Nutrition Standards and Meal Requirements for National School Lunch and Breakfast Programs: Phase I. Proposed Approach for Recommending Revisions

Virginia A. Stallings and Christine L. Taylor, *Editors*

Committee on Nutrition Standards for National School Lunch and Breakfast Programs

Food and Nutrition Board

INSTITUTE OF MEDICINE
OF THE NATIONAL ACADEMIES

THE NATIONAL ACADEMIES PRESS
Washington, D.C.
www.nap.edu

THE NATIONAL ACADEMIES PRESS 500 Fifth Street, N.W. Washington, DC 20001

NOTICE: The project that is the subject of this report was approved by the Governing Board of the National Research Council, whose members are drawn from the councils of the National Academy of Sciences, the National Academy of Engineering, and the Institute of Medicine. The members of the committee responsible for the report were chosen for their special competences and with regard for appropriate balance.

This study was supported by Contract No. AG-3198-C-08-0001 between the National Academy of Sciences and the U.S. Department of Agriculture. Any opinions, findings, conclusions, or recommendations expressed in this publication are those of the author(s) and do not necessarily reflect the view of the organizations or agencies that provided support for this project.

International Standard Book Number-13: 978-0-309-12795-0
International Standard Book Number-10: 0-309-12795-5

Additional copies of this report are available from the National Academies Press, 500 Fifth Street, N.W., Lockbox 285, Washington, DC 20055; (800) 624-6242 or (202) 334-3313 (in the Washington metropolitan area); Internet, http://www.nap.edu.

For more information about the Institute of Medicine, visit the IOM home page at: **www.iom.edu.**

Printed in the United States of America

The serpent has been a symbol of long life, healing, and knowledge among almost all cultures and religions since the beginning of recorded history. The serpent adopted as a logotype by the Institute of Medicine is a relief carving from ancient Greece, now held by the Staatliche Museen in Berlin.

Suggested citation: IOM (Institute of Medicine). 2008. *Nutrition Standards and Meal Requirements for National School Lunch and Breakfast Programs: Phase I. Proposed Approach for Recommending Revisions.* Washington, DC: The National Academies Press.

"Knowing is not enough; we must apply.
Willing is not enough; we must do."
—Goethe

INSTITUTE OF MEDICINE
OF THE NATIONAL ACADEMIES

Advising the Nation. Improving Health.

THE NATIONAL ACADEMIES

Advisers to the Nation on Science, Engineering, and Medicine

The **National Academy of Sciences** is a private, nonprofit, self-perpetuating society of distinguished scholars engaged in scientific and engineering research, dedicated to the furtherance of science and technology and to their use for the general welfare. Upon the authority of the charter granted to it by the Congress in 1863, the Academy has a mandate that requires it to advise the federal government on scientific and technical matters. Dr. Ralph J. Cicerone is president of the National Academy of Sciences.

The **National Academy of Engineering** was established in 1964, under the charter of the National Academy of Sciences, as a parallel organization of outstanding engineers. It is autonomous in its administration and in the selection of its members, sharing with the National Academy of Sciences the responsibility for advising the federal government. The National Academy of Engineering also sponsors engineering programs aimed at meeting national needs, encourages education and research, and recognizes the superior achievements of engineers. Dr. Charles M. Vest is president of the National Academy of Engineering.

The **Institute of Medicine** was established in 1970 by the National Academy of Sciences to secure the services of eminent members of appropriate professions in the examination of policy matters pertaining to the health of the public. The Institute acts under the responsibility given to the National Academy of Sciences by its congressional charter to be an adviser to the federal government and, upon its own initiative, to identify issues of medical care, research, and education. Dr. Harvey V. Fineberg is president of the Institute of Medicine.

The **National Research Council** was organized by the National Academy of Sciences in 1916 to associate the broad community of science and technology with the Academy's purposes of furthering knowledge and advising the federal government. Functioning in accordance with general policies determined by the Academy, the Council has become the principal operating agency of both the National Academy of Sciences and the National Academy of Engineering in providing services to the government, the public, and the scientific and engineering communities. The Council is administered jointly by both Academies and the Institute of Medicine. Dr. Ralph J. Cicerone and Dr. Charles M. Vest are chair and vice chair, respectively, of the National Research Council.

www.national-academies.org

COMMITTEE ON NUTRITION STANDARDS FOR NATIONAL SCHOOL LUNCH AND BREAKFAST PROGRAMS

VIRGINIA A. STALLINGS (*Chair*), The Children's Hospital of Philadelphia, University of Pennsylvania, Philadelphia
KAREN WEBER CULLEN, Children's Nutrition Research Center, Baylor College of Medicine, Houston, TX
ROSEMARY DEDERICHS, Minneapolis Public Schools, Special School District No. 1, Minneapolis, MN
MARY KAY FOX, Mathematica Policy Research, Inc., Cambridge, MA
LISA HARNACK, Division of Epidemiology and Community Health, University of Minnesota, Minneapolis
GAIL HARRISON, School of Public Health, Center for Health Policy Research, University of California, Los Angeles
MARY ARLINDA HILL, Jackson Public Schools, Jackson, MS
HELEN H. JENSEN, Department of Economics, Iowa State University, Ames
RONALD E. KLEINMAN, Massachusetts General Hospital for Children, Harvard Medical School, Boston, MA
GEORGE P. McCABE, College of Science, Purdue University, West Lafayette, IN
SUZANNE P. MURPHY, Cancer Research Center of Hawaii, University of Hawaii, Honolulu
ANGELA ODOMS-YOUNG, Department of Kinesiology and Nutrition, University of Illinois at Chicago
YEONHWA PARK, Department of Food Science, University of Massachusetts, Amherst
MARY JO TUCKWELL, inTEAM Associates, Eau Claire, WI

Study Staff
CHRISTINE TAYLOR, Study Director
SHEILA MOATS, Associate Program Officer
JULIA HOGLUND, Research Associate
SANDRA AMAMOO-KAKRA, Program Associate (until August 2008)
HEATHER BREINER, Program Associate (from August 2008)
CAROL WEST SUITOR, Consultant Writer
LINDA D. MEYERS, Food and Nutrition Board Director

FOOD AND NUTRITION BOARD*

*IOM Boards do not review or approve individual reports and are not asked to endorse conclusions and recommendations. The responsibility for the content of the report rests with the authoring committee and the institution.

Reviewers

This report has been reviewed in draft form by individuals chosen for their diverse perspectives and technical expertise, in accordance with procedures approved by the National Research Council's Report Review Committee. The purpose of this independent review is to provide candid and critical comments that will assist the institution in making its published report as sound as possible and to ensure that the report meets institutional standards for objectivity, evidence, and responsiveness to the study charge. The review comments and draft manuscript remain confidential to protect the integrity of the deliberative process. We wish to thank the following individuals for their review of this report:

George H. Beaton, Department of Nutritional Sciences, University of Toronto
Marilyn Briggs, Center for Integrative Nutrition Environments in School Communities, Department of Nutrition, University of California, Davis
Roger Clemens, University of Southern California School of Pharmacy
Barbara L. Devaney, Human Services Research, Mathematica Policy Research, Inc.
Jean Harris, Government Relations, Pierre Foods
Penny E. McConnell, Food and Nutrition Services, Fairfax County Public Schools, Fairfax, VA
Rodolfo M. Nayga, Jr., Department of Agricultural Economics, Texas A&M University
Barry Sackin, B. Sackin & Associates, L.L.C., Alexandria, VA
Sandra Schlicker, Wellness and Nutrition Services, Office of the State Superintendent of Education, Government of the District of Columbia
Frances H. Seligson, Nutrition Consultant, Hershey, PA
Walter Willett, Department of Nutrition, Harvard School of Public Health

Although the reviewers listed above have provided many constructive comments and suggestions, they were not asked to endorse the conclusions or recommendations nor did they see the final draft of the report before its release. The review of this report was overseen by **Elaine L. Larson,** School of Nursing, Columbia University, and **Johanna T. Dwyer,** Tufts University School of Medicine & Friedman School of Nutrition Science & Policy, Frances Stern Nutrition Center, Tufts-New England Medical Center. Appointed by the National Research Council and Institute of Medicine, they were responsible for making certain that an independent examination of this report was carried out in accordance with institutional procedures and that all review comments were carefully considered. Responsibility for the final content of this report rests entirely with the authoring committee and the institution.

Contents

Summary

Nutrition Standards and Meal Requirements provide the foundation for the National School Lunch Program and the School Breakfast Program, but much has happened since the standards and requirements were last set in 1995. Substantial changes have been made in *Dietary Guidelines for Americans* and in nutrient reference values, and the prevalence of childhood obesity has increased dramatically. This report focuses on how to determine what can be done to help make the meals provided through the National School Lunch Program and the School Breakfast Program more consistent with the current understandings about the diet and health of the children of the United States.

The National School Lunch Program alone now serves more than 30 million children per day. Thus, improvements to the program offer great potential to improve the ability to serve its purpose "as a measure of national security, to safeguard the health and well-being of the Nation's children and to encourage the domestic consumption of nutritious agricultural commodities and other food" (P.L. 79-396). Improvements to the School Breakfast Program would contribute to meeting the same purpose. Together, the two school meal programs can make a great impact because they may provide more than 50 percent of a student's food and nutrient intake on school days. Furthermore, depending on household income, a child may receive program meals at no cost, reduced cost, or full (but a partially subsidized) price. Thus, the programs serve as a safety net for children in need.

When the U.S. Department of Agriculture (USDA) began its school meal programs, nutritional concerns in the United States centered on nutrient deficiencies and underconsumption, and the programs were designed to address those concerns. Although many of the overt nutritional deficiencies in children's diets have largely been eliminated, other nutrition-related concerns have emerged, most notably, a high prevalence of childhood obesity. Although program standards were updated in 1980 and 1995, further revision is needed. The revision of program standards would enable the programs to incorporate public health recommendations and current knowledge about the nutritional needs of children and adolescents. Among the specific reasons for revising the standards are substantial changes in the *Dietary Guidelines for Americans* (which, by law, the school meal programs are required to follow), major changes in nutrient reference values and ways to apply them, and an alarming increase in the prevalence of childhood obesity.

The Nutrition Standards and Meal Requirements provide the foundation for the school meals programs. If the meals offered meet the Nutrition Standards and Meal Requirements in USDA regulations, the USDA subsidizes the cost of the school meals through cash reimbursements. In fiscal year 2007, the value of the cash reimbursements was nearly $10 billion total for both programs. In the same year, USDA also provided the programs with commodity foods valued at approximately $1 billion. The commodity foods available to schools have changed over the years, and states may now choose from a list of more than 180 agricultural commodities, including more foods that are encouraged by *Dietary Guidelines for Americans*, such as fruits and vegetables.

The committee's work has been divided into two phases. This report reflects the outcomes of the Phase I activities. The goal of Phase I was to describe the approach that the Institute of Medicine Committee on Nutrition Standards for National School Lunch and School Breakfast Programs proposes to use in making recommendations for revisions to the Nutrition Standards and Meal Requirements of the school meal programs. During Phase I the committee identified and reviewed available data and information, formulated working principles and criteria, reviewed and assessed the reported food and nutrient intakes by schoolchildren, and described its planning model and analytic methods for developing recommendations for revising the standards. At the time this Phase I report is released, comments from interested parties will be accepted. The report will be discussed during a public forum carried out as part of the next scheduled committee meeting.[1] The input received will be taken into account during the Phase II activities, which will specify the recommendations for revisions.

This Phase I report provides

- an overview of the school meal programs and the participants;
- an overview of reasons for updating program standards;
- the Nutrition Standards and Meal Requirements currently in use;
- topics relevant to updating the Nutrition Standards and Meal Requirements;
- the working principles and criteria that the committee will use to guide its efforts; and
- descriptions of the methods that the committee proposes that it will use to develop recommendations for revisions, including
    - an assessment of the nutrient and food needs of schoolchildren,
    - a planning model that addresses nutrients and foods and the assumptions on which the model is based, and
    - methods for incorporating sensitivity analyses and addressing cost implications and market effects.

Topics related to the competitive foods offered in schools (e.g., foods available in vending machines, at snack bars, and à la carte) are outside the scope of this report.

[1]More information about committee meetings can be found by visiting the IOM website: http://www.iom.edu/fnb/schoolmeals.

CURRENT STANDARDS FOR SCHOOL MEALS

Laws and regulations establish the current Nutrition Standards and Meal Requirements that programs must meet to qualify for cash reimbursement and the receipt of commodity foods from the federal government. Figure S-1 illustrates the steps involved in providing a school lunch or breakfast to a child under the USDA provisions for a reimbursable school meal. The existing planning model is based on the application of the 1995 *Dietary Guidelines for Americans* and the 1989 Recommended Dietary Allowances for selected nutrients averaged over 5 school days. As shown in Figure S-1, the Nutrition Standards set the goals for school meals and the quantitative amounts of foods and nutrients that the meals must provide. Currently, the Meal Requirements allow schools to choose to use either a set of standards associated with a food-based menu planning approach or a set of standards associated with a nutrient-based menu planning[2] approach. Each of these standards encompasses specifications for the amounts of food items or nutrients to be included in the menu planning approach and for the components of a reimbursable meal *as offered* on the cafeteria line and *as served* to the student (based on allowable student selections).

THE COMMITTEE'S TASK

USDA requested that the committee provide recommendations for the updating and revision of the Nutrition Standards and Meal Requirements for the school lunch and breakfast programs. For the phase of the work reported here (Phase I), the committee was asked to (1) outline the proposed criteria and process to be used to develop recommended revisions to the Nutrition Standards and Meal Requirements for both meal programs, (2) discuss how the concepts presented in Institute of Medicine reports and focused on the application of Dietary Reference Intakes to planning and assessment will be applied to school meals in Phase II, and (3) propose plans for undertaking a sensitivity analysis and for considering cost implications and market effects.

WORKING PRINCIPLES AND CRITERIA

The committee developed a set of working principles to focus the committee's deliberations and to guide the committee on the data to be selected and the types of analyses and reviews to be conducted. The committee's working principles are described in Box S-1.

---

[2] USDA often refers to this set of meal standards as nutrient standard menu planning

- Nutrition Standards
  - —Foundation of school meals
  - —Established by USDA and specified in regulation
  - —Nutrient Standards currently reflect required nutrients as calculated quantities for age-grade groups
- Meal Requirements implement the Nutrition Standards
  - —Established by USDA and specified in regulation
- Meal Requirements consist of standards for two types of menu planning approaches
- Menu planning approach is selected by the school food authority and menus are developed at the local level
- Meal—*as offered*—to the student must meet the *as offered* standard for the menu planning approach
- Meal selected by student—*as served*—must meet the *as served* standard for the menu planning approach
- Components of child's meal checked by cashier

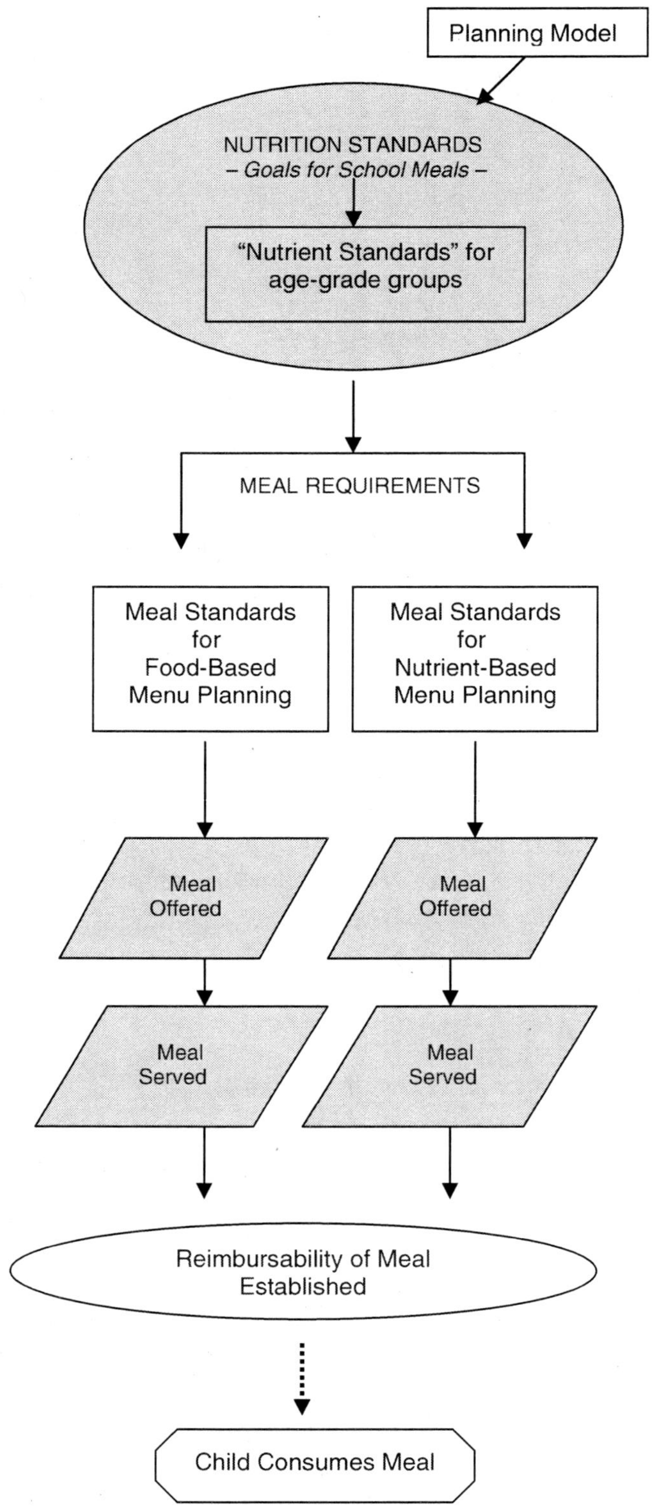

FIGURE S-1 Current path to a nutritious school lunch and breakfast.

BOX S-1
Working Principles for Determining Recommendations for Revisions to the Nutrition Standards and Meal Requirements for School Meals

1. The present and future health and well-being of schoolchildren are profoundly affected by their food and nutrient intakes and the maintenance of healthy body weight.
    a. School meals, when they are consumed, should improve food and nutrient intakes, and those intakes that are inadequate or excessive in schoolchildren should specifically be targeted.
    b. School meals are targeted to children ages 4 through 17 years, but younger children and children of all ages with special needs may be affected by the standards set for the general population.
    c. Recognition will be given to health effects of foods (including beverages) that go beyond those related to their nutrient content.
2. School lunch and breakfast programs, which may contribute to more than 50 percent of the caloric intake by children on school days, offer opportunities to promote the health and well-being of children.
    a. School meals can contribute to beneficial health and dietary patterns and are uniquely positioned to provide a model for healthy meals and to provide opportunities to model and reinforce healthy eating behaviors.
    b. School meals can provide a platform for education in nutrition, environmental responsibility, and food safety.
    c. School meals can be a positive environment for pleasant social interactions.
    d. For children in families characterized by limited resources and food insecurity, school meals provide a critical safety net in meeting their nutritional needs and reducing the adverse effects of food insecurity.
3. School lunch and breakfast programs operate in a challenging and changing environment.
    a. School food service environments (such as facilities, equipment, labor, and skills) are complex and highly varied across the nation as well as from school to school within school districts.
    b. Challenges include the need to meet food safety standards, offer appetizing foods to an increasingly diverse population, adjust to the changes in the available food supply, improve the image and appeal of the program, and achieve a sound financial operation.
    c. Food costs, other direct costs, and indirect costs related to program operation are outpacing the available resources.
    d. In addition to promoting the health and well-being of children, high rates of participation may support the financial stability of school meal programs.
    e. Efforts to change the current school nutrition environments vary, with some districts already making significant strides and others just starting the process of change.
4. Because scientific findings and authoritative recommendations related to the nutrition of children evolve over time, the process of developing recommendations for revisions should be transparent and designed to take into account new evidence-based findings and recommendations.

The committee also developed a proposed set of criteria to be applied during the development of the committee's recommendations for revision of the Nutrition Standards and Meal Requirements. The proposed criteria appear in Box S-2. The committee plans to use iterative processes to derive the recommendations that best meet all four criteria.

BOX S-2
Proposed Criteria for the Nutrition Standards and Meal Requirements for the National School Lunch Program and the School Breakfast Program

Criterion 1. The Nutrition Standards and Meal Requirements are consistent with current dietary guidance and nutrition recommendations to promote health—as exemplified by the *Dietary Guidelines for Americans* and the Dietary Reference Intakes—with the ultimate goal of improving children's diets by reducing the apparent prevalence of inadequate and excessive intakes of food, nutrients, and calories.

Criterion 2. The Nutrition Standards and Meal Requirements will be considered on the basis of age-grade groups that are consistent with the current age-gender categories used for specifying reference values and with widely used school grade configurations.

Criterion 3. The Nutrition Standards and Meal Requirements will result in the simplification of the menu planning and monitoring processes, and they will be compatible with the development of menus that are practical to prepare and serve and that offer nutritious foods and beverages that appeal to students.

Criterion 4. The Nutrition Standards and Meal Requirements will be sensitive to program costs.

APPROACH FOR RECOMMENDING REVISIONS TO THE NUTRITION STANDARDS AND MEAL REQUIREMENTS

The committee's proposed approach to developing recommendations for revisions to the Nutrition Standards and Meal Requirements for the National School Lunch Program and the School Breakfast Program includes the following four steps:

1. applying the working principles to guide the selection of data and the types of analyses and reviews to be conducted and to focus committee deliberations;
2. assessing the dietary intakes of food groups, food subgroups, and nutrients by schoolchildren to identify the food and nutrient intakes of concern for selected age groups;
3. examining various approaches to planning the nutritional aspects of school meals so that the recommendations for revisions to the Nutrition Standards and the Meal Requirements may be effectively incorporated into the requirements for the meals; and
4. applying the criteria shown in Box S-2 in the development of the committee's recommendations for revision of the Nutrition Standards and Meal Requirements. This will include
    a. incorporating sensitivity analysis to study the nutritional impact of the recommended revisions, and
    b. addressing the cost implications and market effects of the recommended revisions.

Therefore, the Phase I work has included an initial assessment of food and nutrient intakes, the development of a proposed planning model, and proposals for incorporating sensitivity analyses and addressing cost implications and market effects.

Review and Assessment of Food and Nutrient Intakes

The committee reviewed and assessed food and nutrient intakes by schoolchildren using national data from USDA sources. Two recently released reports, *The School Nutrition Dietary Assessment Study–III* (SNDA-III) and *Diet Quality of American School-Age Children by School Lunch Participation Status*, which used data from the National Health and Nutrition Examination Survey (1999–2004), provide a comprehensive picture of the diets of U.S. schoolchildren ages 5–18 years. In particular, the committee used data on

- the mean intakes of foods from each of seven MyPyramid food groups plus added fat and sugar (the MyPyramid food guidance system translates the *Dietary Guidelines for Americans* into specific food-based dietary guidance) and
- the distribution of usual intake of calories and of 18 nutrients.

It should be noted, however, that data on dietary supplement intake was not considered since it was not available in the reports used.

Food Group Intakes

The mean daily food group intakes were compared with MyPyramid recommendations for selected calorie levels. The 24-hour usual nutrient intakes were assessed by using the appropriate Dietary Reference Intakes. Mean food group intakes that are below MyPyramid recommendations do not necessarily indicate inadequate nutrient intake, but they do suggest that improvements to the diet would be consistent with current *Dietary Guidelines for Americans* and with relevant Dietary Reference Intakes.

For all children ages 5–18 years, the mean intakes of total vegetables, fruit, whole grains, total meat and beans, and milk were found to be less than the MyPyramid recommendations. The mean vegetable and whole grain intakes were much less than the recommended amounts for all ages, and the mean fruit intake was 50 percent or less than the recommended amounts for children ages 9–18 years. Children consumed larger than recommended amounts of calories from solid fats and added sugars.

Nutrient Intakes

The committee used methods recommended by earlier Institute of Medicine reports to (1) estimate the prevalence of inadequacy of usual nutrient intake or, if applicable, the nutrients with mean and median intake below the Adequate Intake (AI) and (2) identify indications of excessive intake and of usual dietary intakes that exceed the Tolerable Upper Intake Level (UL). The nutrients whose intakes were apparently inadequate varied considerably by age-gender group. Inadequate intakes were the most prevalent among the older children. Among those aged 9 years and older, a high prevalence of inadequate intake was most common for magnesium, vitamin A, phosphorus, zinc, and vitamin C. For adolescent females, the data suggest that the prevalence of inadequate intakes was high for virtually all vitamins and minerals. The prevalence of inadequate intakes may be overestimated for adolescent females, however. In particular, estimated usual nutrient intakes may be substantially lower than actual intakes because studies suggest that underreporting of food intake is common among this group.

Because supplement data were unavailable, it generally was not possible to determine whether nutrients were consumed in amounts that were higher than the UL. For all age groups, however, the prevalence was high for intakes of sodium that exceeded the UL and of intakes of saturated fat that exceeded recommendations in *Dietary Guidelines for Americans*. Zinc intake of more than 25 percent of the children aged 6–8 years exceeded the UL.

The mean and median calcium intakes by older children were less than the AI, and the gap was the highest for adolescents (ages 14–18 years), particularly females. The mean and median intakes of potassium and fiber were substantially less than the AIs for all groups of children. This suggests the potential for inadequate intakes of these nutrients.

Intakes of saturated fat were a major concern. More than three-quarters of the children in all age-gender groups had usual saturated fat intakes that exceeded the recommendation of the *Dietary Guidelines for Americans* of less than 10 percent of total energy. Total fat intake was of less concern: more than 60 percent of the children in all age groups had usual fat intakes that were within the acceptable range. Nonetheless, the usual fat intakes by some children were excessive. More than 90 percent of schoolchildren had usual sodium intakes that exceeded the UL.

Foods and Nutrients Meriting Considerations

As a result of this review and assessment, the foods and nutrients to be given special consideration during Phase II of the study were identified and are listed in Table S-1. The foods and nutrients in this table are those for which a notable proportion of children had intake levels inconsistent with recommended intake levels. The committee will consider them carefully when identifying priority foods and nutrients for the Nutrition Standards and Meal Requirements. In addition, the committee will give special consideration to energy intake for schoolchildren of all ages. Even though reported energy intakes did not appear to be higher than energy requirements, the high prevalence of overweight and obesity (a prevalence of obesity of 17 percent or more, depending on the age and the gender) indicate reason for concern.

The Proposed Planning Model for School Meals

The intent of the planning model is to provide the basis and rationale for developing recommendations for revisions to the Nutrition Standards and Meal Requirements. During Phase I of this study, the committee explored the use of target median intakes (TMIs) to set school meal nutrient targets and the use of USDA MyPyramid food group recommendations as food intake targets. The term *target* is used here to represent a major but preliminary part of the process of setting Nutrition Standards and Meal Requirements for the school meal programs.

A TMI is the median of the usual nutrient intake distribution that would meet the needs of most people in a group. Because the prevalence of inadequate nutrient intakes can be estimated from the percentage of people with usual nutrient intakes that are below the Estimated Average Requirement (EAR), the method of calculating the TMI involves (1) setting a (low) goal for the prevalence of inadequate intakes and (2) calculating how much the current median intake needs to change so that the percentage of people with intakes below the EAR is equal to that goal. The elements of the proposed planning model (setting school meal nutrient targets and food intake targets and combining them) are outlined below.

Proposed Method for Setting Nutrient Intake Targets for School Meals

On the basis of earlier guidance from the Institute of Medicine (IOM, 2003), the committee has proposed seven steps for the setting of nutrient intake targets for school meals.

1. For each age-gender group, determine the target daily energy intake and the goals for the percentages of energy to be provided by breakfast and lunch.
2. For nutrients with an EAR:
    a. Determine the acceptable prevalence of inadequacy and the acceptable prevalence of excessive intakes.
    b. Determine a target nutrient intake distribution to achieve these goals. The median of this distribution is the target median intake (TMI) for the age-gender group.
    c. If necessary, adjust the target nutrient intake distribution so that the prevalence of inadequacy and the prevalence of intakes above the UL are acceptably balanced.
3. For nutrients (other than sodium) with an AI:
    a. Set the TMI equal to the AI for the age-gender group.
    b. If necessary, adjust the TMI to reduce the prevalence of intakes above the UL.
4. For sodium, set the TMI equal to the UL for the age-gender group.

TABLE S-1 Foods and Nutrients Under Consideration in Children's Diets

Age Category	Foods for Which Intakes Are Inadequate, Male and Female	Nutrients for Which Intakes Are Inadequate		Nutrients for Which Intakes Are Excessive[a]	
		Male	Female	Male	Female
Ages 6–8[b]	Fruit Total vegetables Dark green and orange vegetables and legumes Whole grains Total meat and beans Milk	Potassium Fiber	Potassium Fiber	Sodium Saturated fat Total fat Energy[c]	Sodium Saturated fat Total fat Energy[c]
Age 9–13	Fruit Total vegetables Dark green and orange vegetables and legumes Whole grains Total meat and beans Milk	Magnesium Potassium Vitamins A, E Fiber	Calcium Magnesium Phosphorus Potassium Zinc Vitamins A, C, E Fiber	Sodium Cholesterol Saturated fat	Sodium Energy[c] Total fat Saturated fat
Age 14–18	Fruit Total vegetables Dark green and orange vegetables and legumes Whole grains Total meat and beans Milk	Magnesium Potassium Vitamins A, C, E Energy[c] Fiber	Calcium Iron Magnesium Phosphorus Potassium Zinc Vitamins A, C, E, B_6, B_{12} Folate Thiamin Energy[c] Fiber	Sodium Cholesterol Saturated fat Total fat	Sodium Cholesterol Saturated fat Total fat

NOTE: Excessive energy intakes for some age-gender groups may not have been identified because of underreporting.

[a]Excessive amounts of discretionary calories were consumed from solid fat and added sugars; this also constitutes concern relative to recommendations to be made by the committee. Usual intakes of added sugars could not be estimated because relevant data were not available in SNDA-III. The committee notes the quantitative amounts of added sugars in Table 4-5. Furthermore, while intakes of *trans* fatty acids also could not be measured, *trans* fatty acids will be considered as appropriate by the committee during Phase II.

[b]Data for children age 5 years were included in the food intake data.

[c]It is difficult to accurately estimate energy intakes because of under- and overreporting of food intake and a lack of accurate information about customary levels of physical activity.

5. For each nutrient, apply the age-gender TMIs to develop a TMI for each grade category using either a weighted average or a nutrient-density approach.
6. For each nutrient, determine the goal for the percentage of a day's intake to be provided by school breakfast and school lunch, and apply the percentage to the TMI to obtain the school meal nutrient target.
7. Evaluate the proposed school meal nutrient targets in terms of feasibility, cost, and acceptability. Revise the targets as needed to provide an acceptable balance of adequacy, avoidance of excess, feasibility, cost, and acceptability.

The resulting school meal nutrient targets would be consistent with the goals of planning school meals to reduce the prevalence of inadequacy and to reduce the risk of excessive intakes assessed among schoolchildren as described above. However, the impact of changes in the Nutrition Standards and Meal Requirements on children's daily intakes cannot be completely predicted. An intake assessment performed after changes are implemented by USDA would be needed to determine the impact.

Proposed Method for Setting Food Intake Targets for School Meals

The following three steps outline a potentially useful general approach for applying current dietary guidance to the planning of school meals:

1. Select appropriate energy levels.
2. Apply the goal for the percentage of the day's intake (e.g., 20 and 30 percent for breakfast and lunch, respectively) to the MyPyramid food intake pattern for the energy level to obtain amounts of each food group to recommend, that is, the school meal food targets.
3. Consider the recommendations for discretionary calories, which are calories from any source that can be used flexibly (these calories are often from added sugars or solid fats or fat from foods that are not in their lowest-fat form, such as 2 percent fat milk). Staying within these recommendations may require greatly decreasing or eliminating the use of foods that are high in fats and added sugars.

Combining the School Meal Nutrient Targets and Food Targets

Although the committee recognizes the need for nutrient intake targets, the process described above involves many assumptions. Thus, there are many uncertainties about the accuracy of the estimated TMIs. A comparison of the TMIs with the nutrients provided by the MyPyramid food intake patterns shows that adherence to MyPyramid results in diets whose nutrient contents almost always meet or exceed the TMIs. Moreover, adherence to MyPyramid results in diets that are consistent with the *Dietary Guidelines for Americans*. To achieve the planning objectives, the committee will consider recommending that school meal food targets be emphasized in the development of the Nutrition Standards and Meal Requirements for school meals. In particular, the committee may begin by using the MyPyramid food plans as the basis for the school meal targets and then assess projected nutrient intake distributions (using information about the shape of current intake distributions) to determine if the desired objectives are likely to be achieved. As with any method of planning school meals, it would be necessary to assess the children's actual nutrient intakes after changes are implemented to determine if the planning objectives have been achieved.

The school meal food targets would be supplemented with selected school meal nutrient targets for nutrients such as sodium, fat, saturated fat, and cholesterol, and a target for added sugars. If this is workable, this approach may offer an additional advantage: the simplification of meal planning and monitoring.

Proposed Approach for Sensitivity Analysis, Cost Implications, and Market Effects

Sensitivity Analysis

The sensitivity analysis will critically examine each recommendation with respect to likely benefits and consequences. Specifically, the committee will examine the following factors:

1. food intake sample menus with respect to improved adherence to the 2005 *Dietary Guidelines for Americans*,
2. possible effects of nutrient intake contributions from school meals with respect to the prevalence of inadequacy and excessive intake as defined by the Dietary Reference Intakes (DRIs),
3. cost and administrative impacts on food service operations,
4. menu characteristics that influence acceptance by students, and
5. participation rates.

The committee will explicitly state its assumptions and will examine the recommendations relative to each of the factors separately. It will also consider, in a qualitative sense, the net effect of combined benefits and consequences. The committee will examine the recommendations relative to each of the factors separately and consider qualitatively the net effect of the combined benefits and consequences.

Cost Implications

Because USDA does not anticipate that additional funding will be available to schools for implementation of the revised requirements, the committee will aim to design changes in requirements in a manner that keeps program costs economical and as close as possible to current levels (adjusted for inflation). The objective of maintaining program costs at current levels is particularly challenging during a period of rapidly rising food and other costs, as was the case in 2008.

The key sources of information used for examination of the cost implications will be national-level studies of meal and food costs and available publications on the experiences of school districts that have implemented these or similar changes.

Assessment of the impacts of revisions on the costs of reimbursable lunch and reimbursable breakfast meals requires data on the relative amounts of foods used in a representative (typical or average) meal and the relative prices of the individual food items used. The committee proposes to (1) select a representative menu for the lunch and breakfast meals by drawing from menus for each type of meal from frequently observed menus (and food items) from data for elementary schools from the School Nutrition Dietary Assessment Study-III; (2) estimate the cost of the representative menu; and (3) use the representative menu to examine the cost implications of offering the base menu versus those of offering the menus that include the proposed revisions to the school meals offered.

Baseline cost data derived from available food cost data, adjusted to the 2005–2006 school year or more current price levels, will be developed. The adjusted food cost data can be evaluated and calibrated, if necessary, to more recent estimates of the meal costs that are available from the USDA. Although this approach has limitations, it is useful for estimating the cost implications of possible adjustments to the types and amounts of foods needed to meet the recommended revisions to the Nutrition Standards.

Market Effects

The committee will also analyze the economic impacts of its recommendations on school food authorities and on commodity markets. The impact of each of the proposed changes will be included and assessed on the basis of available information. For estimation of the economic effects of its recommendations on commodity markets, the committee will consider the impacts on markets under assumptions of full substitution and full supplementation and the expected levels of substitution and supplementation.

NEXT STEPS

The committee intends to receive input on its proposed approach as described in this Phase I report during a public forum scheduled for January 2009 in Washington, DC (go to http://www.iom.edu/fnb/schoolmeals for details). In addition, interested parties may submit written comments electronically through January 31, 2009, using the following e-mail address: FNBSchoolMeals@nas.edu. If needed and as appropriate in response to the comments that it receives, the committee will consider the need to adjust its approach to developing recommendations for revision of the Nutrition Standards and Menu Requirements for the school meal programs.

This report completes the Phase I activities for this study. The committee's Phase II work will address the development of the recommendations for revision of the Nutrition Standards and Menu Requirements for the School Breakfast Program and the National School Lunch Program. Phase II will culminate in a final report that will also document the scientific information, methods, and assumptions underlying the recommendations. Sensitivity analyses and considerations of cost implications will be integrated with the development of its recommendations. In other words, by applying the four criteria to potential Nutrition Standards and Meal Requirements and then finding a balance among those criteria, the committee will be using a holistic approach to its task. Finally, the Phase II report will include a discussion of the market effects of implementing the revisions that the committee recommends.

1

Introduction

The National School Lunch Program (NSLP) and the School Breakfast Program (SBP) are large and important child nutrition programs overseen by the U.S. Department of Agriculture (USDA). The department has requested that the Institute of Medicine (IOM) of the National Academies review and recommend revisions to the Nutrition Standards and the Meal Requirements that are currently used to plan these school meals. Under the auspices of the Food and Nutrition Board of the IOM, an expert committee was convened to study the issues and make recommendations.

This committee has undertaken the study in a two-phase process. This report, which describes Phase I of the study, focuses largely on the development of plans that will be used to make sound recommendations for the revision of the Nutrition Standards and Meal Requirements. Topics related to the competitive foods offered in schools (e.g., foods available in vending machines, at snack bars, and à la carte) are outside the scope of this report. Throughout the report, children and adolescents in the United States who are of school age (4–18 years) are referred to as "schoolchildren."

Chapter 1 includes background information about the school meal programs and reasons that revisions in standards and requirements are needed. Chapter 2 provides detailed information about the current Nutrition Standards and Meal Requirements. Chapter 3 covers the committee's working principles and study criteria and then introduces the approach that it plans to use to develop its recommendations. Chapter 4, which addresses the first step in the committee's approach, provides an overview of the food and nutrient needs of schoolchildren. Chapter 5 presents the committee's proposed planning model for the approach to be used to develop Nutrition Standards, and Chapter 6 describes analyses that will be conducted in the course of developing final recommendations. Appendix A identifies the many abbreviations, acronyms, and specific terms that are included in this report.

This introductory chapter provides an overview of the NSLP and the SBP, addresses the reasons that the Nutrition Standards and the Meal Requirements for these programs need to be updated and revised, describes the committee's task, and briefly summarizes findings from a selection of large-scale evaluations that the committee may need to consider as it develops recommended revisions to the standards.

OVERVIEW: PROGRAMS AND PARTICIPANTS

Operating under the aegis of the Food and Nutrition Service of USDA, the NSLP and the SBP play key roles in ensuring the nutrition and health of children in the United States. The NSLP offers nutritious lunches in 99 percent of U.S. public schools and in 83 percent of private and public schools combined (USDA/ERS, 2004). The SBP offers breakfasts in approximately 85 percent of public schools (USDA, 2007a). With about 95 percent of U.S. children eating one or two meals at school on school days (including children who bring their lunches from home), the school cafeteria holds the potential to promote sound dietary habits among all schoolchildren, regardless of whether they participate in the school meal programs (Kennedy and Davis, 1998).

Purpose, Brief History, and Description of the Programs

Purpose

The purpose of the NSLP, as summarized in the enabling legislation, is "as a measure of national security, to safeguard the health and well-being of the Nation's children and to encourage the domestic consumption of nutritious agricultural commodities and other food" (*National School Lunch Act*, P.L. 79-396, Stat. 281 (June 4, 1946): §2). This section of the National School Lunch Act has not been changed over the life of the program—more than six decades. Congress authorized the SBP as a pilot program in 1966 (*Child Nutrition Act*, P.L. 89-642, (October 11, 1966)). When Congress permanently authorized the SBP in 1975 under an amendment to the Child Nutrition Act (P.L. 94-105, (October 7, 1975)), it stated "it is the purpose and intent of the Congress that the school breakfast program be made available in all schools where it is needed to provide adequate nutrition for children in attendance" (Martin, 2008a).

Brief History—Federal Reimbursement Linked to Regulations

From the onset, federal reimbursement for school meals has been linked to specific regulations. The NSLP was required to operate on a nonprofit basis and to serve meals at no cost to children who were determined to be unable to pay (*National School Lunch Act*, P.L. 79-396, Stat. 281 (June 4, 1946): §2). In addition, Section 9 of the National School Lunch Act gave the Secretary of Agriculture the authority to prescribe the minimum nutritional requirements for school lunches. In 1946, the secretary prescribed three food-based meal patterns (USDA, 2008a):

1. Type A lunches, which consisted of 8 ounces of whole milk, 2 ounces of protein-rich food, ¾ cup of vegetables or fruit, one portion of a bread product, and 2 teaspoons of butter or fortified margarine;
2. Type B lunches, which had the same specification for bread and milk and half the portion of the other food groups as Type A lunches and which were devised for schools where facilities were not available to provide a Type A lunch; and
3. Eight ounces of whole milk, which supplemented lunches brought from home.

The SBP initially had a meal pattern similar to that of the Type A school lunch but was adapted for a smaller meal size (Martin, 2008b). Meals that conformed to the meal patterns were eligible for some degree of federal reimbursement. Initially, the federal reimbursement for meals was much lower than their cost (Martin, 2008b).

Laws and regulations governing the school meal programs have evolved over the years (see Appendix B). Much of the basis for the current Nutrition Standards and Meal Requirements is a function of work undertaken by USDA in 1995 and known as the School Meals Initiative for Healthy Children (SMI) (USDA, 1995), as well as legislation passed by Congress in 1996 (*Personal Responsibility and Work Opportunity Reconciliation Act of 1996,* P.L. 104-193 (August 22, 1996): §702).

Brief Program Description

Currently, the school meal programs must provide meals at no cost (free) or at a reduced-price for children certified by the school food authorities to be eligible for them. Others may purchase the meals at full price. Schools must offer meals whose food components are consistent with program regulations, but a meal qualifies for federal reimbursement even if a student accepts fewer food items, as long as the number of items meets the minimum specified by the *as served* standard (*National School Lunch and Child Nutrition Act Amendments,* P.L. 94-105, 1975). Current USDA subsidies for the cost of these meals are described in detail in Chapter 2.

As illustrated in Figure 1-1, the current standards and requirements comprise many elements. As a first step, a planning model guides the development of the Nutrition Standards and Meal Requirements. The current planning model uses the 1995 *Dietary Guidelines for Americans* (HHS/USDA, 1995) and the 1989 Recommended Dietary Allowances (RDAs) (NRC, 1989), as prescribed by law. USDA established specific minimum standards for the levels of calories, protein, vitamins A and C, calcium, and iron as well as specified levels of calories from total fat and saturated fat to be included in school meals[1] (USDA, 1995). These specifications now constitute the Nutrition Standards for school meals. As part of the Nutrition Standards specification, calculations are carried out to develop the quantitative amounts of nutrients for relevant age-grade groups. These calculated amounts are currently referred to as "nutrient standards." The right-hand side of Figure 1-1 shows how the elements are connected to provide a pathway to a nutritious school breakfast or lunch. The child's consumption of the foods he or she has selected is shown at the end of the path. Consumption of the food is a key part of ensuring the health of children, but it is out of the direct control of the meal's providers. However, standards will be most effective if they result in nutritious foods that appeal to children. The left-hand side of the figure provides a brief description of each of the elements. The standards and requirements outlined in Figure 1-1 are described in detail in Chapter 2.

---

[1]Although there is not a required mandate for the levels of sodium, cholesterol, and dietary fiber in school meals, the amounts of these nutrients are required to be calculated in the nutrient analysis as carried out by school food programs and state agencies during SMI reviews.

- Nutrition Standards
  - —Foundation of school meals
  - —Established by USDA and specified in regulation
  - —Nutrient Standards currently reflect required nutrients as calculated quantities for age-grade groups

- Meal Requirements implement the Nutrition Standards
  - —Established by USDA and specified in regulation

- Meal Requirements consist of standards for two types of menu planning approaches

- Menu planning approach is selected by the school food authority and menus are developed at the local level

- Meal—*as offered*—to the student must meet the *as offered* standard for the menu planning approach

- Meal selected by student—*as served*—must meet the *as served* standard for the menu planning approach

- Components of child's meal checked by cashier

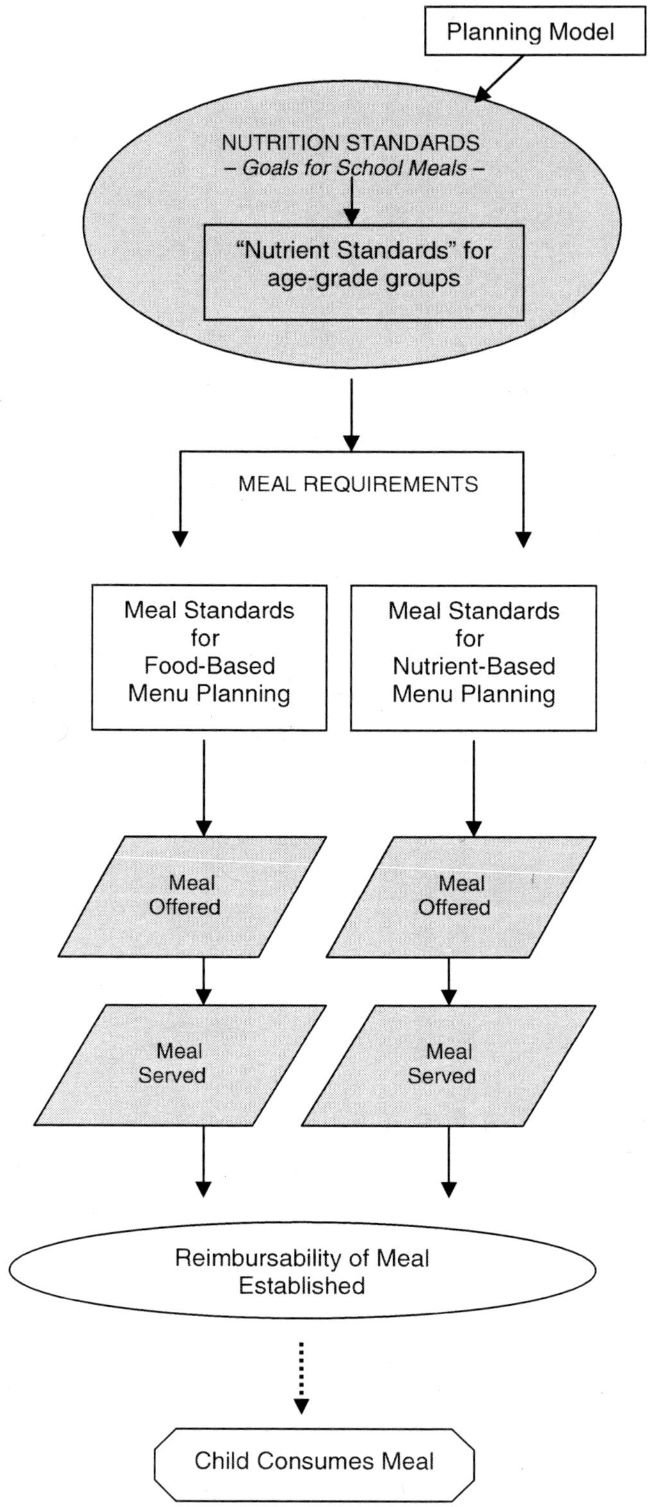

FIGURE 1-1 Current path to a nutritious school lunch and breakfast.

For this report, the general term "standards" is occasionally used and is intended to be a comprehensive term for the Nutrition Standards and Meal Requirements. In the case of Meal Requirements, the "meal standards" for each of the menu planning approaches encompass the specifications for the amounts of the food items (food-based menu planning) as well as the specifications for the food components or menu items that are designated for a meal *as offered* and for a meal *as served.*

Program Size and Student Participation

The potential reach of the school meal programs is very large: during the 2005–2006 school year, more than 49.1 million children were enrolled in U.S. public schools (U.S. Department of Education, 2007). If a school participates in one or both of the school meal programs, any child who attends the school may obtain the school meal. On average, about 60 percent of children in schools that offer school meals eat a school lunch (USDA, 2007a). In fiscal year (FY) 2007, an average of 30.6 million schoolchildren participated in the NSLP on each school day. About 24 percent of children in schools that offered the SBP participated in the program, on average, equaling 10.1 million children each school day. In FY 2007, the participating schools served about 5.1 billion lunches at a cost of approximately $8.7 billion to USDA and 1.7 billion breakfasts at a cost of $2.2 billion to USDA (USDA/ERS, 2008).

Figure 1-2 shows how the average rate of student participation in the NSLP and the SBP has changed over the past 40 years. The sharp dip in student participation that occurred between 1981 and 1982 was triggered by provisions in the Omnibus Reconciliation Act of 1981 (P.L. 97-35, Stat. 95 (August 13, 1981): §357–933) that substantially reduced financial support for the school meal programs and resulted in a decrease in the number of students purchasing lunches at full price. From 1985 to 2000, the rate of growth in school lunch participation was about equal to the rate of growth in school enrollment (USDA, 2008b).

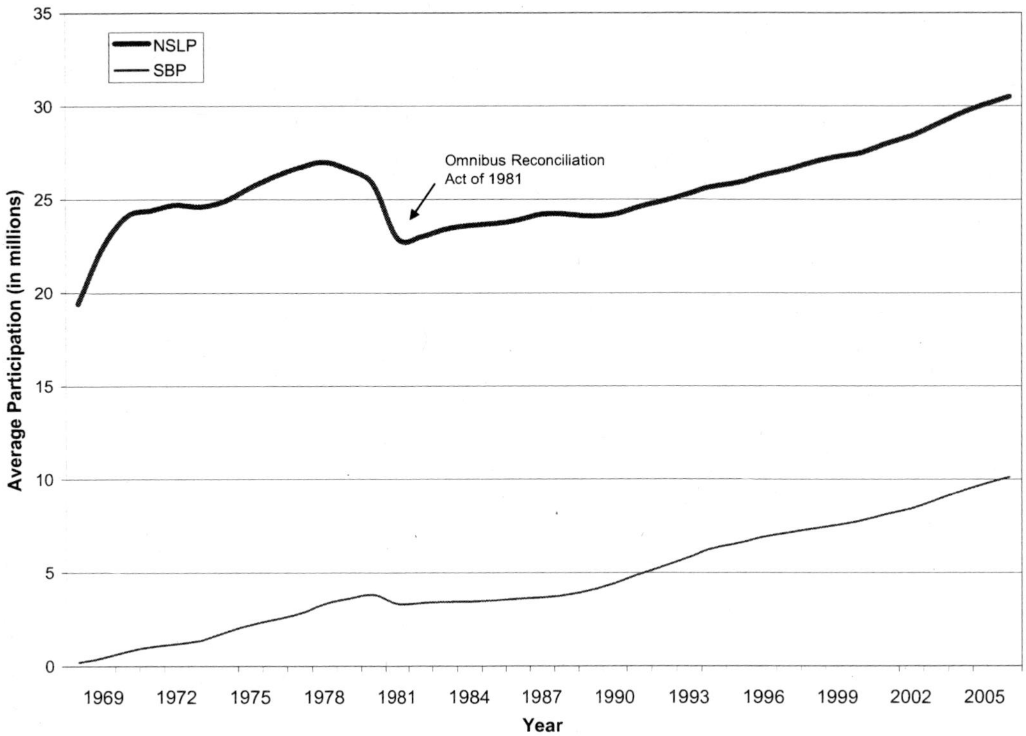

FIGURE 1-2 Change in average student participation in the National School Lunch Program and the School Breakfast Program, 1969–2007.
SOURCE: USDA, 2008c,d.

Diversity of the School Population

The U.S. school-age population is highly diverse both across the nation and within many individual schools. Table 1-1 shows the distribution of enrollment in public schools by race and ethnic background for fall 1995 and fall 2005. Notably, diversity is increasing: the Hispanic and Asian/Pacific Islander populations are growing at a rapid rate.

TABLE 1-1 Distribution of Enrollment in Public Schools by Race and Ethnic Background, Fall 1995 and Fall 2005

	Percent Enrollment				
Year	White	Black	Hispanic	Asian/Pacific Islander	American Indian/ Alaska Native
1995	64.8	16.8	13.5	3.7	1.1
2005	57.1	17.2	19.8	4.6	1.2

SOURCE: U.S. Department of Education, 2008a.

Differences in the racial and ethnic compositions of school districts in different parts of the United States are not readily revealed by the information in Table 1-1. However, Figure 1-3 illustrates the diversity present in the five largest school districts in the 50 states during the 2005–2006 school year.

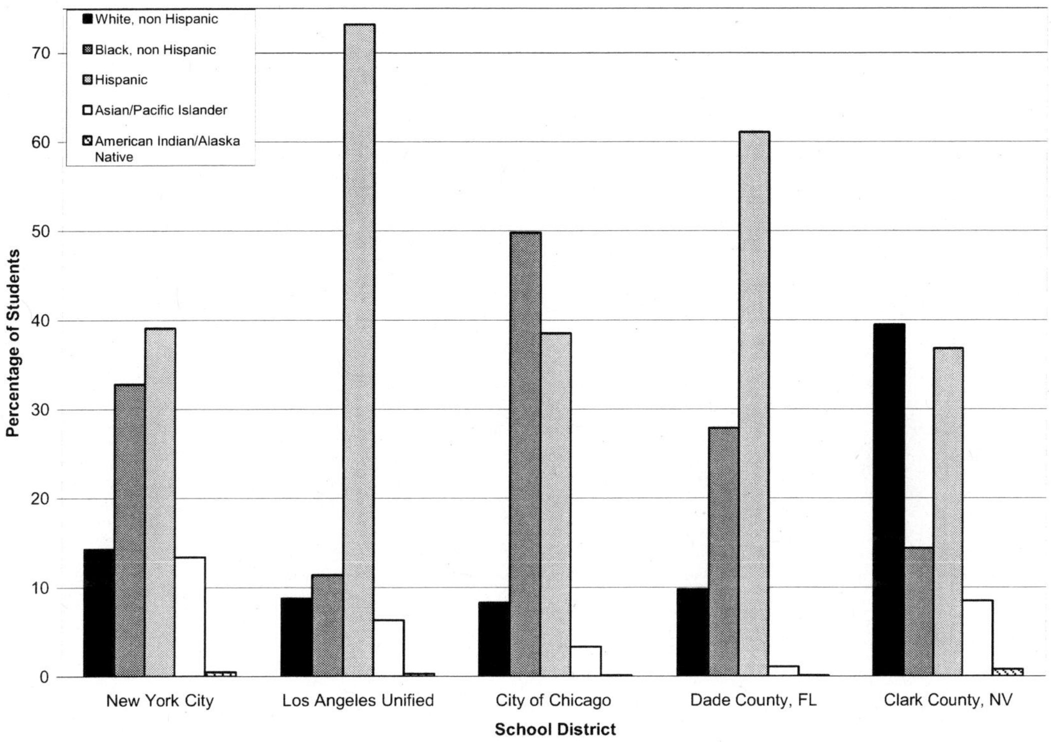

FIGURE 1-3 Racial and ethnic compositions of public elementary and secondary schools in the five largest school districts of the 50 states.
SOURCE: U.S. Department of Education, 2008b.

Immigration is likely responsible for a portion of the changes shown in Table 1-1 and will probably contribute to future changes (U.S. Department of Education, 2000a). Data from the 2006 Annual Social and Economic Supplement to the Current Population Survey indicate that, for all children under the age of 18 years, about 21 percent have a foreign-born parent or parents, are foreign-born themselves, or both (U.S. Census Bureau, 2006).

Low-Cost Meals for Schoolchildren

The school meal programs provide children with access to nutritious, low-cost food to support their growth, development, and health. Both the NSLP and the SBP can provide a safety net for children in need, given the provisions that make school meals available free or at a reduced cost to eligible participants. If the child lives in a household whose income is at or below 130 percent of the federal poverty level (or if the household receives food stamps,[2] Temporary Assistance for Needy Families, or assistance from the Food Distribution Program on Indian Reservations), the child is eligible for a free school lunch and a free school breakfast. The McKinney-Vento Homeless Assistance Act (P.L. 100-77, 1987), as amended by the No Child Left Behind Act (P.L. 107-110, 2001), states that students who are identified by a school district as homeless or highly mobile automatically qualify for free meals and do not need to complete the full application process (U.S. Department of Education, 2004).

If the household income is between 130 percent and 185 percent of the poverty level, the child is eligible for a reduced-price meal (USDA, 2008b). Ordinarily, children from households with incomes over 185 percent of the poverty level pay full price. Even full price meals, however, are subsidized by the government to a small extent through both cash reimbursements and the provision of USDA food commodities (see School Food Purchasing Data Illuminate the Usage of Major Types of Food later in this chapter and USDA Commodities in Chapter 2).

Figures 1-4 and 1-5 show the changes in student participation from 1969 to 2007 by payment type for the NSLP and the SBP, respectively. For the NSLP, the *percentage* of students obtaining meals in the full-price category has decreased over time (USDA, 2008c).

---

[2]As of October 1, 2008, the new name for the Food Stamp Program is the Supplemental Nutrition Assistance Program (SNAP).

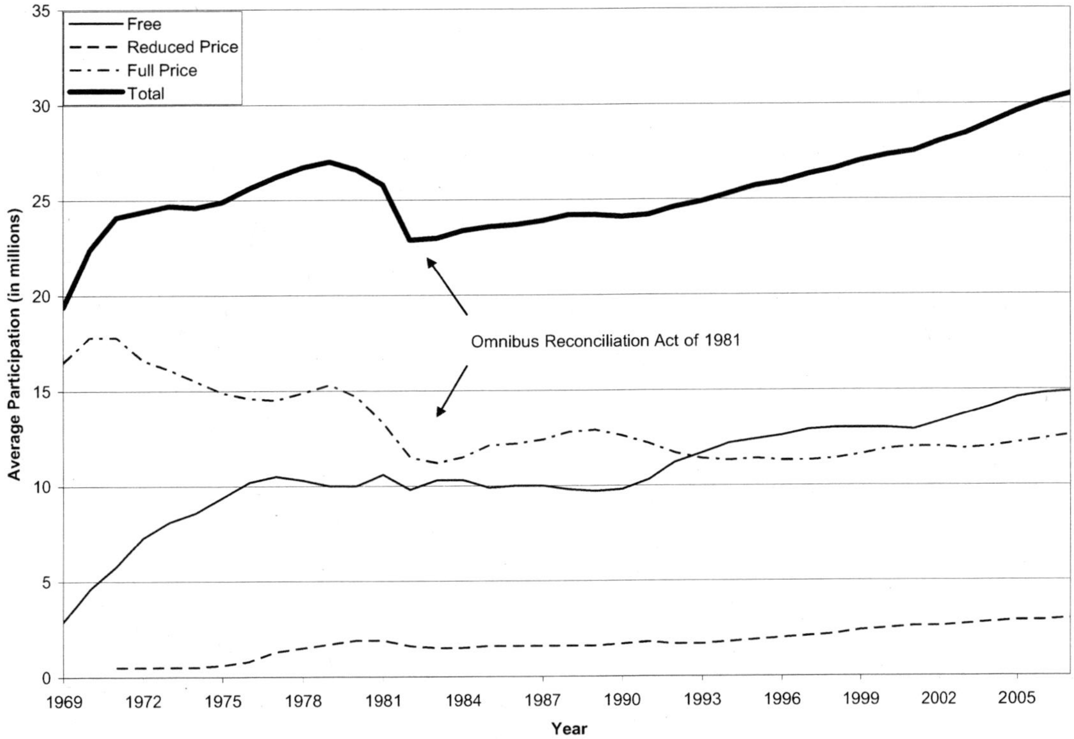

FIGURE 1-4 Change in student participation in the NSLP by meal cost category, 1969–2007. SOURCE: USDA, 2008c.

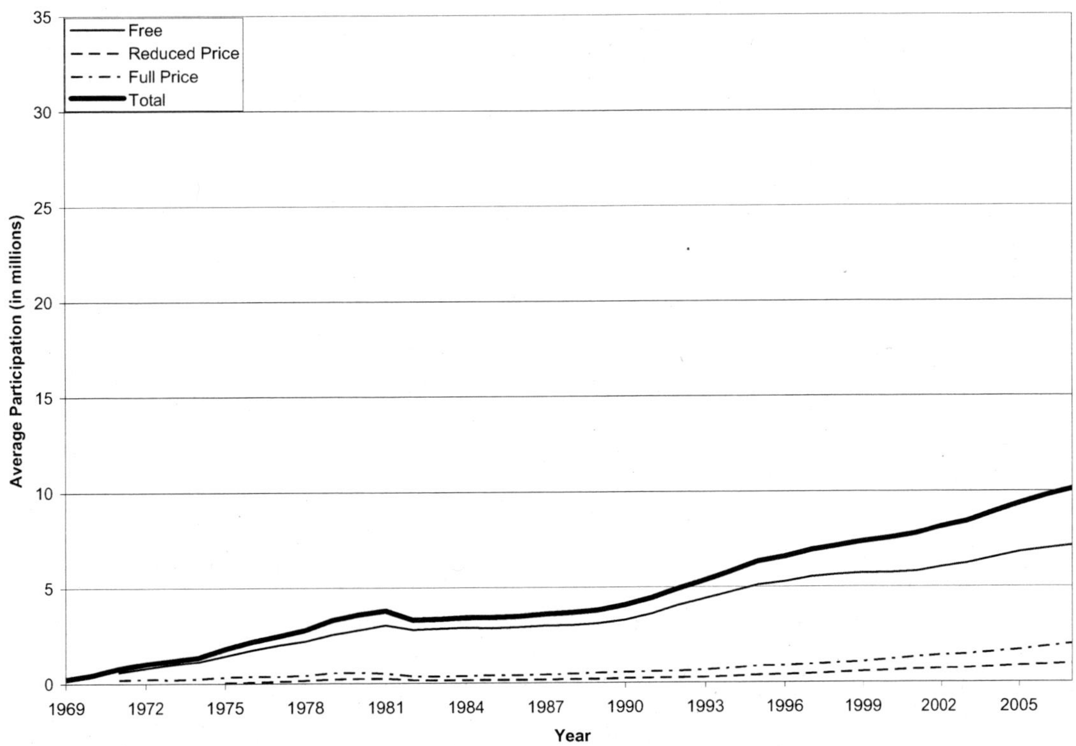

FIGURE 1-5 Change in student participation in the SBP by meal cost category, 1969–2007. SOURCE: USDA, 2008d.

Currently, more children receive free meals than meals in the other two price categories. On average, 59 percent of the NSLP lunches served in FY 2007 were served to students who received their meals free or at a reduced price (USDA, 2008c). In the SBP, 81 percent of the meals were served free or at a reduced price (USDA, 2008d). Notably, approximately 10 percent of schools now serve breakfast free of charge to any child who wishes to participate (universal-free breakfast) (SNA, 2007).

Given the current provisions, children who participate in both the NSLP and the SBP are offered at least 58 percent of the 1989 RDAs (NRC, 1989) for selected vitamins and minerals (at least 25 percent at breakfast and 33 percent at lunch). Thus, for the 36 weeks, on average, that children are in school, school meals may be the source of more than 40 percent of their weekly intakes of these nutrients. Therefore, school meals clearly have the potential to make a valuable contribution to the food intake and nutritional health of children, especially if their other meals and snacks are of poor nutritional quality or are unavailable.

WHY IS THERE A NEED FOR UPDATING AND REVISIONS?

Congress has recognized the need to update and revise the Nutrition Standards and Meal Requirements for the school meal programs. In 2004, Congress passed the Child Nutrition and WIC[3] Reauthorization Act (P.L. 108-265), which required USDA to issue guidance and regulations to promote the consistency of the standards for school meal programs with the standards provided in the most recent *Dietary Guidelines for Americans* and the Dietary Reference Intakes (DRIs) (IOM, 1997, 1998, 2000a, 2001, 2002/2005, 2005).

Reasons for the current call for updates and revisions are shown in Box 1-1. The first two bullets in Box 1-1 represent the major reasons that Congress called for the revisions.

BOX 1-1
Rationale for the Call to Revise the Current Nutrition Standards and Meal Requirements

- Current Nutrition Standards and Meal Requirements are inconsistent with current *Dietary Guidelines for Americans*, especially with regard to meeting recommended intakes within energy needs by following a balanced meal pattern; increasing intake of fruits, many types of vegetables, and whole grains; minimizing intake of *trans* fat; a 25 to 35 percent range of total fat intake as a percentage of calories, limiting sodium intake to 2,300 mg per day.[a]
- They are inconsistent with current nutrient reference values and were developed without the benefit of new understandings regarding how such values should be applied in assessing and planning diets for groups of people.
- They may be contributing to the increased prevalence of childhood obesity in the United States.
- Their implementation poses challenges for many school food operators.

[a]See Appendix C for specifics.

[3]WIC is the Special Supplemental Nutrition Program for Women, Infants, and Children.

The last major change to the standards and requirements for school meals went into effect in 1995 (see Appendix B). Since then, authoritative dietary guidance and recommended nutrient intakes have changed, the prevalence of obesity has increased substantially, and stakeholders have voiced concerns and implemented some initiatives for change.

Some of the relevant developments and changes that have occurred since 1995 are discussed below.

Dietary Guidelines for Americans Has Changed

Dietary Guidelines for Americans, first issued in 1980 (HHS/USDA, 1980) and revised every 5 years since then, provides the public with authoritative guidelines on diet and health. Moreover, according to law (*National Nutrition Monitoring and Related Research Act*, P.L. 101-445 (October 22, 1990): §301), these guidelines form the basis of federal food, nutrition education, and information programs, including the school meal programs. Currently, the Nutrition Standards for school meals reflect the applicable recommendations of the 1995 *Dietary Guidelines for Americans*. The recommendations provided in the latest edition of *Dietary Guidelines for Americans*, issued in 2005 (HHS/USDA, 2005), are more extensive and specific than those presented in 1995, as shown in more detail in Appendix C. Furthermore, many of the key elements of the most recent nutrient reference values—Dietary Reference Intakes (DRIs), issued between 1997 and 2005—are incorporated in the 2005 *Dietary Guidelines for Americans*, as discussed in the text below.

Reference Values for Nutrients Have Changed

Public law and regulations enacted in the mid-1990s specified the use of the 1989 RDAs (NRC, 1989) to set the nutritional parameters for the NSLP and the SBP (USDA, 1994a). However, beginning in 1997 and continuing through 2005, the IOM developed an expanded set of reference values called the DRIs (IOM, 1997, 1998, 2000a, 2001, 2002/2005, 2005). In addition to more specifically incorporating chronic disease end points into considerations of the establishment of DRIs, the DRIs differ from the 1989 RDAs, in that

- DRIs cover a more extensive list of nutrients, one of which is fiber;
- DRIs include several types of reference values in addition to the RDAs, including Estimated Average Requirements (EARs), Adequate Intakes (AIs), Tolerable Upper Intake Levels (ULs), and Acceptable Macronutrient Distribution Ranges (AMDRs) (see Chapter 5 for further details);
- DRIs use different age-gender groups, different units for vitamins A and E, and a different method for handling estimated energy needs; and
- The DRI process established recommendations concerning total fat and saturated fat, as recommendations for those two nutrients were not available in 1989.

The IOM also developed methods for the use of the EARs, AIs, ULs, and AMDRs to assess nutrient intakes by particular groups of individuals (IOM, 2000b) and to plan intakes for particular groups (IOM, 2003). Such changes are relevant to the task of making recommendations to revise the school meal programs. Notably, the use of RDAs for assessing or planning intakes for groups of people is no longer recommended.

The Prevalence of Obesity Among Schoolchildren Has Increased

Much concern has been raised about the increasing prevalence of obesity among U.S. children, as indicated by the age- and gender-specific body mass indexes (BMIs) at the 95th percentile or higher (CDC, 2008a). Between 1976 and 2006, striking increases in the percentages of obese children occurred, as shown in Figure 1-6.

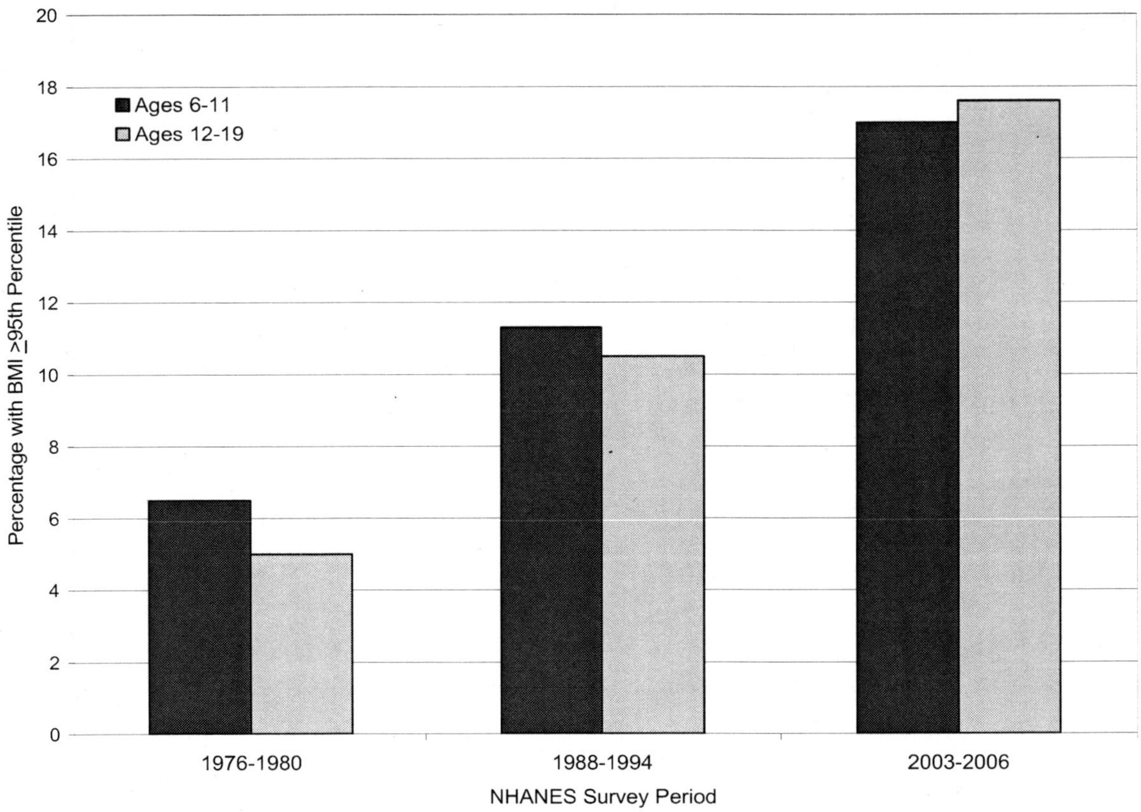

FIGURE 1-6 The increasing prevalence of obesity (BMIs ≥95th percentile of Centers for Disease Control and Prevention growth charts, calculated as weight [in kilograms] divided by height [in meters squared]) among schoolchildren, 1976–2006.
NOTE: NHANES = National Health and Nutrition Examination Survey.
SOURCES: CDC, 2008a; Ogden et al., 2008.

Table 1-2 presents recent data on three categories of high BMIs among U.S. children. Notably, nearly one-third of all children are overweight or obese (BMI ≥85th percentile). Specifically, close to 17 percent of children are obese and another 16 percent are overweight. In all three BMI categories and for each age group, the prevalence is higher among males than among females and is higher among non-Hispanic blacks and Mexican Americans than among non-Hispanic whites (data not shown) (Ogden et al., 2008).

Despite the limitations in the use of BMI as a measure of pediatric obesity (Ebbeling and Ludwig, 2008), the prevalences of obesity shown in Table 1-2 indicate that large numbers of children and adolescents are at increased risk for chronic disease: type II diabetes (Messiah et al., 2008), hypertension (Jago et al., 2006), and metabolic syndrome (De Ferranti et al., 2006) in the short term and cardiovascular disease in the long term (Baker et al., 2007).

TABLE 1-2 Prevalence of High BMIs Among U.S. Children, by Age, 2003 to 2006

Age group, yr (both genders)	Percentage of children (SE) with the Following BMIs according CDC Growth Charts:		
	≥97th Percentile	≥95th Percentile	≥85th Percentile
6–11	11.4 (0.9)	17.0 (1.3)	33.3 (2.0)
12–19	12.6 (1.0)	17.6 (1.2)	34.1 (1.5)

NOTE: Data come from the National Health and Nutrition Examination Survey (NHANES). Pregnant adolescents were excluded. Values for BMIs were rounded to one decimal place. CDC = Centers for Disease Control and Prevention; SE = standard error.

SOURCE: Derived from Ogden et al., 2008. Reprinted, with permission, from Journal of the American Medical Association. May 28, 2008. 299(20):2403.

No studies have been found that link the school meal programs with obesity. However, because of the substantial contribution of school meals to total intake, revision of the Nutrition Standards and Meal Requirements might hold potential for reducing the possible contribution of the school meal programs to childhood obesity.

Stakeholders Are Calling for Change

Concomitantly with the developments mentioned above, stakeholders have actively sought to make changes to the school meals programs. The committee held an open meeting with representatives from professional organizations, associations, the food industry, and state and county agencies and food service operations at which the participants shared information and viewpoints concerning the need for revision to the Nutrition Standards and Meal Requirements for the school meal programs (Appendix D provides the workshop agenda). Several associations have initiatives that include actions to promote the application of the 2005 *Dietary Guidelines for Americans* to school meals. An important emphasis of food service operators and representatives of the food industry is that the recommendations for change need to be feasible and that cost, ease of preparation and service, and acceptance of the foods by the students be considered. They also encouraged authorities to make changes on a gradual basis.

In addition to calling for revision of the Nutrition Standards and Meal Requirements, the *Child Nutrition and WIC Reauthorization Act of 2004* (P.L. 108-265: §204) mandated that local wellness policies be developed in all school districts by the 2006–2007 school year. As a result, the level of involvement at the local level (by parents, students, representatives of the school food authority, the school board, the school administrator, and other members of the public) has increased substantially. Thus, additional calls for change are originating at the local level

THE COMMITTEE'S TASK

To help respond to the Congressional requirement that USDA issue new guidance and regulations for the Nutrition Standards and Menu Requirements of the school meal programs, the USDA has sought the assistance of the Institute of Medicine (IOM) to provide recommendations to update and revise the nutrition- and food-related standards and requirements for the school lunch and breakfast programs. The last revisions to these meal programs took place in 1995. The specific charge to the committee is shown in Box 1-2.

BOX 1-2
Charge to the Committee

- Specify a planning model for school meals (including targets for intake) as it may relate to nutrients and other dietary components for lunch and breakfast;
- Recommend revisions to the Nutrition Standards and, in consideration of the appropriate age-grade groups for schoolchildren, provide the calculations that quantify the amounts of nutrients and other dietary components specified in the Nutrition Standards;
- Recommend the Meal Requirements necessary to implement the Nutrition Standards on the basis of two existing types of menu planning approaches (i.e., the food-based menu planning [FBMP] approach and the nutrient-based menu planning [NBMP] approach); for this task, the committee was asked to recommend Meal Requirements that include
    - standards for a food-based reimbursable meal by identifying
        - the food components for *as offered* and *as served* meals and
        - the amounts of food items per reimbursable meal by age-grade groups and
    - standards for a nutrient-based reimbursable meal by identifying
        - the menu items for *as offered* and *as served* and
        - the 5-day average amounts of nutrients and other dietary components per meal; and
- Illustrate the practical application of the revised Nutrition Standards and Meal Requirements by developing menus for a 4-week cycle that will meet the recommended standards for the age-grade groups.

The committee's work has been divided into two phases. For the phase of the work reported here (Phase I), the committee was asked to identify and review the available data and information, formulate criteria, carry out an assessment of the food and nutrient intakes by schoolchildren, and describe its planning model and the analytic methods that it plans to use to develop recommendations for revising the standards. As specified in the committee's task, at the time that this Phase I report is released, comments from interested parties will be accepted and the report will be discussed during a public forum carried out as part of the next scheduled committee meeting.[4] The input received will be taken into account during the Phase II activities, which will specify the recommendations for revisions.

The committee's overall task is to review and assess the food and nutritional needs of schoolchildren in the United States on the basis of the 2005 *Dietary Guidelines for Americans* (HHS/USDA, 2005) and the DRIs and to use that review as a basis for recommending revisions to the Nutrition Standards and Meal Requirements for the NSLP and the SBP. As part of its task, the committee has been asked to consider the critical issues described in Appendix E. The goal is

[4]More information about committee meetings can be found by visiting the IOM website for this study: http://www.iom.edu/fnb/schoolmeals.

the development of a set of well-conceived, practical, and economical recommendations that reflect current nutrition science, increase the meals' contents of the key food groups (as appropriate), improve the ability of the school meal programs to meet the nutritional needs of children, foster healthy eating habits, and safeguard children's health.

Furthermore, the request to the committee specifies that the recommendations be designed to be economical and keep program costs as close as possible to current levels adjusted for inflation. The committee intends to identify recommendations based on the best available nutrition science and will take cost into account.

Finally, current law requires the programs to provide meals containing one-third of the RDA for lunch and one-fourth of the RDA for breakfast. This language was adopted before the new conceptual approach related to DRIs was developed and could be incorporated into legislation. Therefore, this Phase I report describes the planned approach to use DRIs and the Phase II report will compare differences (with examples and rationale) between basing standards on the RDA approach and basing the standards on the DRI methodology.

RELEVANT FINDINGS FROM LARGE-SCALE EVALUATIONS OF SCHOOL MEAL PROGRAMS

The committee has conducted an initial examination of large-scale evaluations of school meal programs to identify information that may be useful in revising the Nutrition Standards and Meal Requirements. Beginning in 1983, USDA funded numerous large-scale studies to evaluate the school meal programs and selected components of the programs (Appendix F). The topics of the evaluations have included the nutrient contents of the meals, the effects of the meals on the participants' nutritional status, operational issues, and costs. The studies not only identified a number of strengths of the programs but also identified a number of areas for improvement.

This section provides a brief summary of findings that the committee may review as it considers possible revisions it will propose. During Phase II, the committee will conduct targeted literature searches to determine whether additional studies may provide information useful to the process of developing recommendations for revisions to the Nutrition Standards and Meal Requirements.

School Nutrition Dietary Assessment Studies Provide Data on Program Compliance and Students' Intake

All three studies in the School Nutrition Dietary Assessment (SNDA) series, SNDA-I (USDA, 1993), SNDA-II (USDA, 2001a), and SNDA-III (USDA, 2007a) provide data on the extent to which schools were in compliance with standards that were current at the time. All three studies showed that the lunches provided through the NSLP provided one-third or more of the 1989 RDAs for the required vitamins, minerals, and nutrients and that the breakfasts provided through the SBP provided one-fourth or more of the RDAs, on average.

Based on data collected from nearly 400 elementary, middle, and high schools during the 2004–2005 school year (USDA, 2007a), compliance with the standards for key nutrients ranged from 71 percent for energy to more than 98 percent for calcium and protein. Compliance for cholesterol and dietary fiber exceeded 90 percent. However, all the lunches exceeded the sodium recommendation and few met the standards for total fat (19 percent) and saturated fat (28 percent). In the same study, compliance with current standards was less favorable for the SBP.

While nearly 66 percent of schools met the standard for vitamin C, less than 50 percent of schools met the standards for protein, vitamin A, calcium, and iron. Less than 25 percent of schools offered meals that complied with the standards for energy and total fat, and less than 10 percent complied with the saturated fat standard.

The three SNDA studies also indicate change over time. SNDA-II (1998–1999 school year) found that school meals were lower in fat, on average, than they had been in 1991–1992 (SNDA-I) and that the percentage of schools that met the Nutrition Standards for total fat and saturated fat in meals *as offered* had increased from about 0 percent to 15 to 20 percent. SNDA-III (2004–2005 school year) found no increase in the percentage of schools serving lunches that met the Nutrition Standard for total fat compared with the percentage found in SNDA-II but a significant increase in the percentage of schools that met the Nutrition Standard for saturated fat. In all three SNDA studies, breakfast was more likely than lunch to meet the dietary recommendation for total fat. On average, school lunches and school breakfasts remain high in sodium.

Revenues Cover Reported Costs but Not Full Costs

Using reported costs (not necessarily actual total costs), both the 1994 and the 2008 cost studies (USDA, 1994b, 2008e) found that school food authorities operated at a break-even level, on average. Reimbursable lunches generated a revenue surplus that many schools used to offset SBP losses, and in some cases, the surplus was used to reduce losses from non-program-related food services, such as à la carte food services. Notably, however, revenues fell short of covering full costs. The reported costs often excluded such costs as indirect costs, equipment depreciation, utilities, fuel (for off-site delivery), all of which contribute to the full cost. Revenues covered about 92 percent of reimbursable meals but only 61 percent of nonreimbursable meals (à la carte food services, adult meals, food services from vending machines, and catering) (USDA, 2008e).

Nutrient-Based Menu Planning Poses Challenges but Offers Flexibility

The Nutrient Standard Menu Planning approach (called Nutrient-Based Menu Planning for the purposes of this report) is described in more detail in Chapter 2. The two evaluations of this menu planning approach (USDA, 1997, 1998a) revealed a number of challenges related to staff resources, time requirements, and the software used but reported that the approach offered increased flexibility in menu planning. The resulting menus tended to be lower in total fat and saturated fat than they were before this approach was initiated and had comparable abilities to meet the RDAs. The rates of student participation in the meal programs and costs remained about the same.

School Food Purchasing Data Illuminate the Usage of Major Types of Food

The School Food Purchasing Study (USDA, 1998b) obtained national estimates of food purchases made in the 1996–1997 school year by public school districts participating in the NSLP and the SBP. That study included all food purchases, not only those that related to reimbursable meals served under the NSLP and the SBP. Other food purchases may have included à la carte foods, foods for staff meals, and foods served though USDA food assistance programs (Child and Adult Care, Summer Food Services, and the Nutrition Program for the Elderly).

On the basis of the findings of that study, in the 1996–1997 school year, school districts purchased 83 percent of their food commercially, received 13 percent of their food as donated commodities, and obtained 4 percent of their food in the form of processed foods containing donated commodities. The five leading food categories in terms of total value of the food donated were fluid milk, pizza, ground beef, cheese, and potato products. USDA donations were the primary source of the supply of peanuts and peanut butter, turkey products, beef products, vegetable oils and shortening, cheese, flour, and eggs. In an examination of purchasing practices, no one method produced the best cost per pound for all food items.

Since the 1984–1985 school year, there had been large changes in the use of a number of foods, as briefly summarized below.

- Higher rates of use: Breakfast cereals, prepared foods, yogurt, and fruit drinks
- Lower rates of use: Fluid milk, butter, salad dressing, vegetable oils and shortening, lard, and other animal fats (consistent with recommendations to reduce total and saturated fat in meals)
- Increased volumes: Fresh fruits and vegetables, with a much larger variety of these foods being donated

Higher Calorie Level and Universal-Free School Breakfast Program Increase Program Participation

The first evaluation of the School Breakfast Program (USDA, 1998c) found that the calorie content of breakfast affects participation. In particular, when the standards for breakfast specify that the meal is to contain a level of calories greater than 10 percent of the RDA, the likelihood that low-income elementary school students will eat breakfast increases. In a more recent 3-year pilot study (USDA, 2004), a universal-free school breakfast program resulted in a substantial increase in school breakfast participation (for all children), especially in the schools that served breakfast to students in the classroom.

The School Meals Initiative Has Led to Several Operational Improvements

The School Meals Initiative (SMI) aims to achieve far-reaching reform of the school meal programs relative to upgrading the nutritional content of school meals. It was finalized as a regulation in 1995 (USDA, 1995). The three SMI implementation studies (USDA, 2000a, 2001b, 2002a) addressed operational topics but not the extent to which schools met the SMI standards. In particular, the three SMI studies showed increasing and substantial progress in the implementation of menu planning approaches. In the 1999–2000 school year, nearly two-thirds of all school districts reported that they had fully implemented their chosen approach to menu planning, and many more were far along in the process. Menu changes, if any, tended to be modest, however. The SMI implementation studies found that the percentage of school districts that adopted nutrient-based menu planning remained stable at about 25 percent, but there was evidence that those that used this system of menu planning became more efficient at doing so. Nonetheless, key elements of nutrient-based menu planning (entering and analyzing recipes, entering and analyzing menus, and obtaining missing nutrient information) have remained challenging for many districts. The Team Nutrition Pilot Study (USDA, 1999), which preceded the SMIs, provided some data on how broad-scale nutrition education efforts may positively affect children's food consumption behaviors, including the acceptance of menu choices.

Salad Bars Are More Prevalent in the Upper Grades and in Affluent Schools

A review of salad bars in schools (USDA, 2002b) was based on SNDA-II data collected during the 1998–1999 school year. The review found that salad bars are more likely to be available in high schools than in elementary schools and in more affluent schools than in schools with a high percentage of children who receive free or reduced-price meals. Schools with salad bars may offer a wider variety of vegetables and fruits than other schools. The presence of a salad bar was associated with student participation in the NSLP in middle and high schools, but the study lacked data with which it could be determined whether the salad bars increased participation rates or with which the quantities of fruits and vegetables served to or consumed by students could be estimated.

Few Peer-Reviewed Studies Address Program Impact

Literature searches for relevant publications in peer-reviewed journals has not yet identified large-scale studies using data collected after the implementation of the SMI in 1995, the date of the most recent change in the Nutrition Standards and Meal Requirements. Gleason and Suitor (2003) used data from the 1994–1996 Continuing Survey of Food Intakes by Individuals to examine the impact of participation in the NSLP on children's dietary intake at lunchtime and over 24 hours. By controlling for selection bias with a fixed-effects model, the investigators found that the NSLP was associated with an increased 24-hour intake of calcium, magnesium, phosphorus, zinc, vitamin B_{12}, riboflavin, and fiber. Participants had lower intakes of added sugars than did non-participants, but higher intakes of total fat and saturated fat. In earlier peer-reviewed studies that used SNDA data, NSLP participation was positively related to the intake of selected nutrients at lunch (Burghardt et al., 1995; Gordon et al., 1995) and to daily dietary fat intake; but the other effects of program participation on 24-hour intakes were smaller, and fewer findings were statistically significant (Burghardt et al., 1995).

IMPLICATIONS

The NSLP and the SBP have a long and impressive history of providing nutritious low-cost meals to schoolchildren. Over time, efforts have been made to update the programs' Nutrition Standards and Meal Requirements to keep pace with the changing understandings of children's nutritional needs. There have been major developments in dietary guidance and nutrient reference standards and their application to programs since the last major revisions to the Nutrition Standards and Meal Requirements. It is now time to develop recommendations for further revisions to the Nutrition Standards and Meal Requirements of the school meal programs so that the program can achieve greater benefits for the nation's children.

Chapter 2 helps to clarify the nature of the charge to the committee by describing the current standards that are the subject of the committee's review and subsequent recommendations, along with topics that may be important to the committee as it considers recommendations.

2

The Nutrition Standards and Meal Requirements: Description and Topics Relevant to Their Revision

Laws and regulations establish the specifications that those schools participating in the National School Lunch Program (NSLP) and the School Breakfast Program (SBP) must meet to qualify for cost reimbursement from the federal government. The nutritional specifications, currently provided as Nutrition Standards and Meal Requirements, were designed to ensure nutritious meals for schoolchildren, and they have evolved over time (see Appendix B). An understanding of the current U.S. Department of Agriculture (USDA) provisions for school meals sets the stage for the consideration of recommendations for revising the current standards and requirements. This chapter outlines the Nutrition Standards, Meal Requirements, and related components of the current NSLP and SBP. The chapter also covers topics that the committee identified to be important to its considerations, many of which also were identified as critical issues by USDA (see Appendix E).

CURRENT NUTRITION STANDARDS AND MEAL REQUIREMENTS

The Nutrition Standards provide the foundation for the NSLP and the SBP. The related Meal Requirements facilitate the actions needed to implement the Nutrition Standards and develop menus and meals. At present, Meal Requirements reflect two sets of meal standards. The food-based menu planning (FBMP) approach focuses on the types and the amounts of foods to be offered. The second set of meal standards, the nutrient-based menu planning (NBMP) approach makes use of computer software to plan menus that meet the Nutrition Standards. Local school food authorities (SFAs) decide which menu planning approach is to be used and, hence, which set of meal standards is to be followed. The SFAs then develop their specific menus accordingly. Currently, approximately 70 percent of schools use the FBMP approach (USDA, 2007a). The Nutrition Standards and Meal Requirements (and their related sets of meal standards) are described further in sections below.

To receive federal reimbursement for the meal, SFAs must first offer a meal that meets the *as offered* and reimbursable meal standard for the menu planning option that the school has chosen to follow. Next, the student must select the items that are consistent with the *as served* reimbursable meal standard. On the basis of prescribed record-keeping requirements, SFAs may claim federal reimbursement for the meal. However, the level of reimbursement depends on whether the individual student qualifies for a full-price, reduced-price, or free meal. This is described in further detail in the "Meal Requirements" section below.

Figure 2-1 identifies the standards that are the main focus of the committee's task and illustrates their interrelationships. The task includes the specification of standards for the two types of menu planning approaches currently encompassed within the Meal Requirements (these current standards are listed in detail in Appendixes G and H). In addition, to make appropriate recommendations, the committee was asked to articulate an approach (a planning model) for the development of the Nutrition Standards that is consistent with the current *Dietary Guidelines for Americans* and with current applications of existing nutrient reference values.

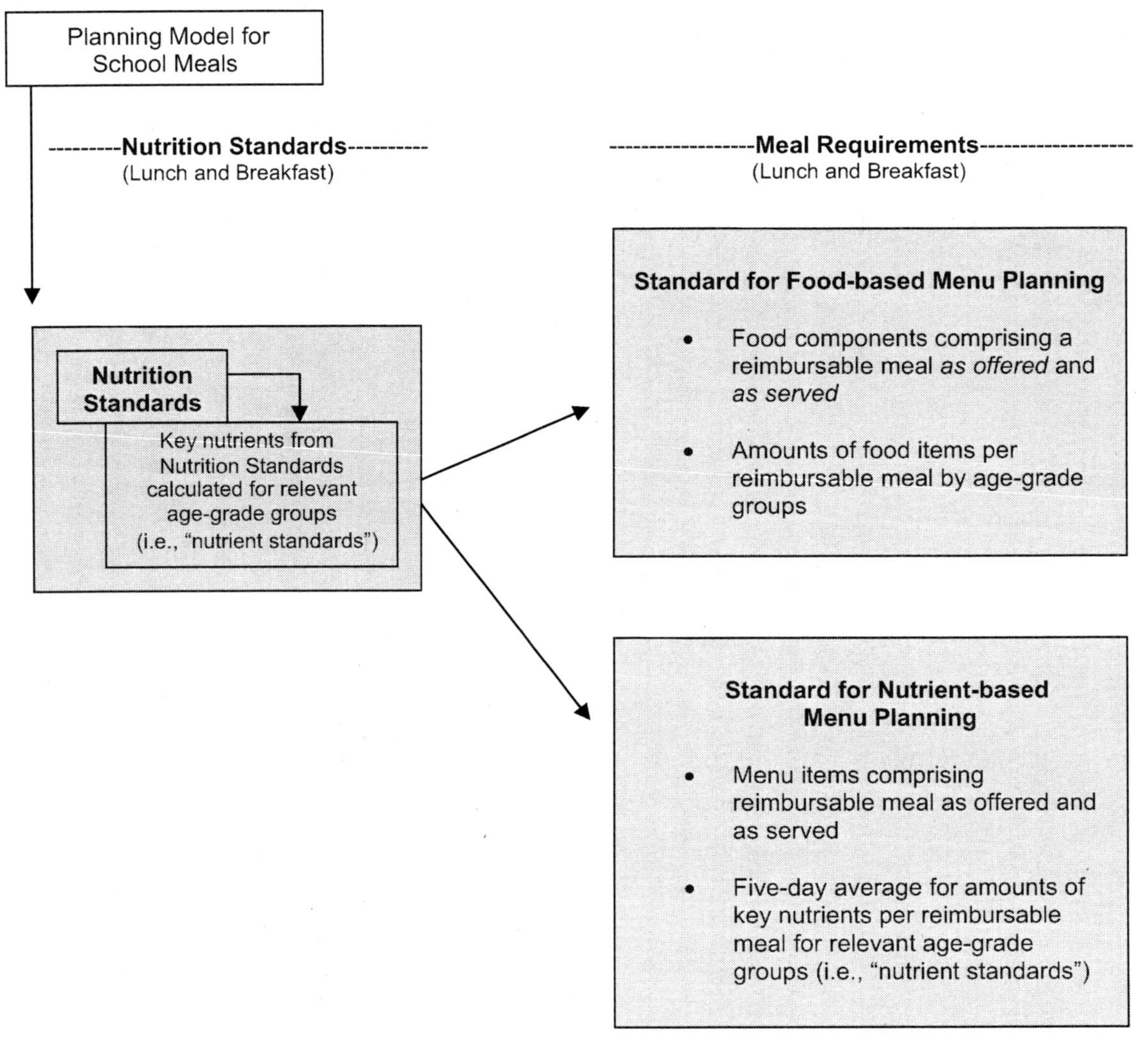

FIGURE 2-1 Current standards for school lunch and breakfast under review by the committee.

Nutrition Standards for School Meals

Description of the Current Nutrition Standards

The existing Nutrition Standards (Table 2-1) were put in place in 1995 through a policy initiative and related regulation known as the School Meals Initiative (SMI) for Healthy Children (USDA, 1995). This 1995 USDA regulation requires that the meal programs comply with the then current *Dietary Guidelines for Americans* and that school lunches and breakfasts provide at least one-third and one-fourth of the 1989 Recommended Dietary Allowances (RDAs) (NRC, 1989) for selected nutrients, respectively, on a daily basis, as averaged over 5 consecutive school days. In addition, the program regulations specify the maximum amounts of total fat and saturated fat and the minimum number of calories.[1] Legislation passed in 1996 (*Personal Responsibility and Work Opportunity Reconciliation Act of 1996,* P.L. 104-193, (August 22, 1996)) mandated that school lunch and breakfast provide, on average over a 5-day week, one-third and one-fourth of the RDAs, respectively.

TABLE 2-1 Current Nutrition Standards for the National School Lunch and Breakfast Programs[a]

Nutrient	Standard for the Meal	
	School Lunch	School Breakfast
Key nutrients		
•Calories	⅓ of the REA[b,c]	¼ of the REA[b,c]
•Protein	⅓ of the RDA[c]	¼ of the RDA[c]
•Calcium, iron, vitamins A and C	⅓ of the RDA[c]	¼ of the RDA[c]
•Total fat	≤30% of calories	≤30% of calories
•Saturated fat	<10% of calories	<10% of calories
Recommended but not required		
•Cholesterol and sodium	Decrease levels in the meals	
•Dietary fiber	Increase level in the meals	
•Grain products, vegetables, and fruits	Increase levels in the meals	
•Eat a variety of foods		

[a]These standards apply to the average content of meals over one school week (5 days).
[b]REA = Recommended Energy Allowance (NRC, 1989).
[c]These reflect the minimum standard for the appropriate age-grade group.
SOURCE: USDA, 1995.

[1]The term "calories" is used to refer to kilocalories throughout this report.

In addition to calories, the existing Nutrition Standards focus on protein, calcium, iron, and vitamins A and C because of the roles that these nutrients play in promoting growth and development (USDA, 1995). These five nutrients were intended to serve as a practical proxy to ensure that school meals include other essential nutrients. The components of the Nutrition Standards that address total fats and saturated fats support the recommendations in the 1995 *Dietary Guidelines for Americans* (HHS/USDA, 1995), as do the recommended (but not required) levels of cholesterol, sodium, and dietary fiber. All 11 of these nutrients and other dietary components are identified on the nutrition labels of food products, providing an important source of information for school menu planners.

As part of its task to recommend revisions to the Nutrition Standards, the committee was asked to specify a planning model, that is, to describe and provide a rationale for the approach used to establish the Nutrition Standards. The existing planning model for Nutrition Standards is based on application of the 1995 *Dietary Guidelines for Americans* and the 1989 RDAs for selected nutrients, as averaged over 5 school days.

Many terms are associated with the Nutrition Standards. The term *Nutrition Standards* itself reflects the comprehensive list of the overall dietary goals of interest, regardless of whether they are currently required or only recommended by USDA. The required components of the Nutrition Standards are called *key nutrients.*[2] The term *nutrient standards* is familiar to many who work with the school meal programs and refers to those quantitative values that specify the amounts of the key nutrients for the age-grade groups[3] (on a 5-day average). The calculations on which these amounts are based are described later in this chapter. The nutrient standards are incorporated directly into the NBMP approach (Appendix H). For FBMP, however, the nutrient standards were used in developing the specifications for the meal standards[4] that reflect the food components and amounts in the Meal Requirements (Appendix G), and SFAs may use the nutrient standards as a measure when monitoring the quality of the menus they have planned.

Furthermore, some have used the term *indicator nutrients* to refer to those key nutrients that serve as a useful proxy for major food groups and for identifying dietary patterns that are likely to include a range of essential nutrients. Vitamin C, for example, if it is present in an adequate amount in food sources, is likely to indicate the presence of important amounts of certain other vitamins and trace elements. Recently, the term *nutrients of concern* (or, sometimes, *indicators of concern*) has been used to refer to nutrients for which current levels of consumption may be problematic (e.g., calcium). Nutrients of concern are not specified within current USDA provisions for school meals, but one or more of the key nutrients may be nutrients of concern.

Calculation of Amounts of Key Nutrients for Age-Grade Groups (Nutrient Standards)

The Nutrition Standards specify that the lunch meal contain one-third of the 1989 RDA for key nutrients and that the breakfast meal contain one-fourth of the 1989 RDA for key nutrients. However, the Nutrition Standards must be quantified in a manner that tailors the amounts for the age-grade groups receiving the school meal—for example, children in a school for grades 7–12, all of whom receive meals from a single cafeteria line. For several nutrients, this quantification

---

[2]Practitioners have tended to informally refer to the key nutrients as divided into two groups: So-called leader nutrients (calories, protein, calcium, vitamin A, vitamin C) and *Dietary Guidelines for Americans* nutrients (the percentage of calories from total fat and the percentage of calories from saturated fat).

[3]As used in the school meal programs, *age-grade groups* actually are designated by grades, such as kindergarten through grade 3.

[4]These standards are often referred to as meal patterns.

involves the use of weighted RDAs. The use of weighting allows the determination of a single representative value when children in the age-grade group have different RDAs on the basis of their age and gender. These calculated values have been called *nutrient standards;* but, to avoid unnecessary confusion, this report incorporates these values into the broader term *Nutrition Standards*. From this point forward in the report, the term *Nutrition Standards* is used to encompass the general list of nutrients and other dietary components, including the quantities calculated for each age-grade group.

Table 2-2 shows the amounts of nutrients that are to be provided to schoolchildren on the basis of the current Nutrition Standards and as specified for relevant age-grade groups. These amounts are based on a 5-day average. Therefore, over the course of a school week, the average nutrient content per meal must be consistent with these amounts. The age-grade groups included in Table 2-2 are those specified for the various menu planning approaches that are described in the "Meal Requirements" section below. Different menu planning approaches incorporate different age-grade groups.

TABLE 2-2 Current Nutrition Standards: Amounts of Nutrients That Are to Be Provided to Children, by Age-Grade Group[a,b]

	Lunch					Breakfast		
Food Component	Preschool	K–3	K–6	Grades 4–12[c]	Grades 7–12	Preschool	K–12	Grades 7–12
Calories	517	633	664	785	825	388	554	618
Fat (% of kcal)	≤30	≤30	≤30	≤30	≤30	≤30	≤30	≤30
Saturated fat (% of kcal)	<10	<10	<10	<10	<10	<10	<10	<10
Protein (g)	7	9	10	15	16	5	10	12
Calcium (mg)	267	267	286	370	400	200	257	300
Iron (mg)	3.3	3.3	3.5	4.2	4.5	2.5	3.0	3.4
Vitamin A (RAE)	150	200	224	285	300	113	197	225
Vitamin C (mg)	14	15	15	17	18	11	13	14

NOTE: g = grams; K = kindergarten; kcal = kilocalories (or calories, as used in this report to refer kilocalories); mg = milligrams; RAE = retinol activity equivalents.

[a]These amounts are also referred to as "nutrient standards."

[b]The preschool group is used in all menu planning approaches, the K–3 group is used in the traditional food-based approach and is optional in the enhanced food-based and nutrient-based approaches, the K–6 group is used in the enhanced food-based and nutrient-based approaches, the grade 4–12 group is used in the traditional food-based approach, and the grade 7–12 group is used in enhanced food-based and nutrient-based approaches and is optional in the traditional food-based approach. Menu planners are encouraged to use smaller age-grade groupings to better meet the nutritional needs of students. At a minimum, they must use the established grade groups (e.g., the K–6 and 7–12 groups) or the other grade options (e.g., the preschool and K–3 groups). School food authorities (SFAs) can modify the age-grade groups to reflect the grades within that SFA. If one age-grade is outside the established range of the K–6 or the grade 7–12 group, the school may use the age-grade group in which the majority of children fit. If more than one age-grade is outside the range, an SFA must use two menus and the relevant calculated quantities as specified by the Nutrition Standards.

[c]The SFA or school always has the option of serving the meal appropriate for the grade 4–12 age-grade group for all students in the school district or school under the traditional food-based approach for lunch.

SOURCE: Derived from USDA, 2000b, 2008f.

Meal Requirements

School menu planners have some flexibility to plan nutritious and appealing meals that vary from day to day, but these meals must provide the required components of the Nutrition Standards on a daily basis, as averaged over the school week (Table 2-2). These standards, as specified by USDA, guide the menu planning process. The term *Meal Requirements* refers to the set of meal standards used to develop menus and meals so as to implement the Nutrition Standards. The meal standards are specific to the type of menu planning process used (the FBMP approach or the NBMP approach) and are delineated in Appendixes G and H.

Menu Planning Approaches

The two menu planning approaches and related meal standards serve several important purposes. In particular, they

- facilitate meal planning,
- enable local SFAs to decide what specific foods they will serve,
- help ensure that the Nutrition Standards will be met over the course of the 5 consecutive days of the school week, and
- enable local SFAs to serve meals that qualify for reimbursement.

Characteristics of the FBMP and the NBMP approaches are summarized in Table 2-3. Aspects of the Meal Requirements that are specific to each approach are indicated by gray shading.

Food-based menu planning approaches There are two food-based approaches, the traditional and the enhanced approaches. The first two columns of Table 2-3 show that the traditional food-based approach is similar to the enhanced food-based approach but that the enhanced food-based approach uses a larger number of servings of vegetables and fruits and of grains and breads at lunch. It also uses different age-grade groups (see the rows Reimbursable lunch [as offered standard] and Age-grade groups: Lunch). The *as served* standard for a reimbursable breakfast is the same for both the traditional and the enhanced FBMP approaches.

Nutrient-based menu planning approaches The two NBMP approaches (nutrient standard menu planning and assisted nutrient standard menu planning) are the same and appear together in the rightmost column of Table 2-3. Both approaches develop menus utilizing a computerized process to ensure that the nutrient content conforms to the standards. The NBMP approach is implemented by the use of USDA-approved computer software for nutrient content analysis. Either the SFA itself or (with assisted planning) an outside source uses the software to plan and analyze menus. The state agency must approve the initial cycle menus, recipes, and other pertinent information, such as food specifications.

Alternative approaches A fifth option (not shown) is known as the alternative menu planning approach or as any reasonable approach, as cited in regulation (*Healthy Meals for Children Act,* P.L. 104-149 (May 29, 1996): § 9). It allows states and school districts to develop their own approaches, but these are subject to the requirements established in the USDA regulations.

Comparison of the Approaches

For the NBMP approaches, the meal standards regarding the nature of the menu items are relatively broad (e.g., at a minimum, a lunch must contain an entrée, fluid milk, and a side dish). The actual number of menu items required each day depends on the number needed to meet the Nutrition Standards averaged over a week. In contrast, schools using the FBMP approaches must meet portion size specifications for all the food components in the lunch menu (namely, fluid milk, meat or meat alternate, vegetable or fruit, and grains or bread). The portion size specifications used in the FBMP approach differ somewhat by age-grade group, as shown in Appendix G.

On the basis of data from the third School Nutrition Dietary Assessment (USDA, 2007a), approximately 48 percent of the schools that offer lunch use the traditional food-based method of menu planning, 22 percent use the enhanced food-based method, and 30 percent use a version of the nutrient-based method.

Offer Versus Serve

Under existing requirements, schools must *offer*—that is, make available on the cafeteria line—the menu items that on a daily basis comprise a reimbursable meal. The "offer versus serve" (OVS) provision, which was mandated by law for senior high school lunch programs in 1976 (USDA, 1976) and currently is a widely used option for lower grades, introduced a new standard: the *as served* standard for reimbursable meals. As shown in Table 2-3 under both menu planning approaches, the *as offered* standards are distinct from *as served* standards for meals. For schools that take part in OVS, a student may select—that is, be *served*—fewer menu items than the number that must be offered, but the selected menu items must match those required under the OVS provisions (i.e., meet the *as served* meal standard shown in Table 2-3 for a reimbursable meal). Although students may decline specified foods, the cost (if any) of the meal to the student stays the same. It should be noted that a meal *as served* does not necessarily equate to what a student may actually consume. For schools that do not take part in OVS, the *as offered* standard applies.

Finally, in regard to Meal Requirements overall, the SMI calls for periodic (usually every 5 years) reviews of a school's meal program. The goal is to promote adherence to the standards and to provide the technical assistance that may be needed. The SMI reviews are carried out by the state authorities, and at times they are assisted by USDA staff. Key elements of the review include analysis of a week's set of menus for nutrient content, the school's implementation of the age-grade group specifications, and validation that the school is serving the meal as planned (personal communication, R. Orbeta, Food and Nutrition Service, USDA, September 2008).

Although Table 2-3 provides a general overview of the components of the current Meal Requirements, the committee must address the specific meal standards within the Meal Requirements. The current meal standards for the FBMP approach are presented in Appendix G, and those for the NBMP approach appear in Appendix H.

TABLE 2-3 Characteristics of Menu Planning Approaches for School Meals[a]

Characteristic	Food-Based Menu Planning Approach[b]: Traditional Approach	Food-Based Menu Planning Approach[b]: Enhanced Approach	Nutrient-Based Menu Planning (Nutrient Standard Menu Planning or Assisted Nutrient Standard Menu Planning) Approach[c]
How meals are planned and evaluated	Food components and food items/Nutrient content analysis	Same as traditional approach	Nutrient content analysis; must contain minimum required menu items
Food components, food items, and menu items offered	Minimum quantities as established for food components and food items (see Appendix G)	Same as traditional approach	Menu items as established by the menu planner to meet the Nutrition Standards calculated for age-grade groups (see Appendix H)
Computer hardware and software	• Not required • State agency will conduct nutrient analysis on SMI review	Same as traditional approach	• Menu planning is based on nutrient content analysis • The SFA or school must have hardware and USDA-approved software and use nutrient content analysis to plan meals to meet the Nutrition Standards calculated for the age-grade group or use an outside source for assistance with analysis of the appropriate Nutrition Standards before reimbursable meals are served
Reimbursable lunch (*as offered* standard)[d]	A minimum of five food items in specific quantities must be offered from the following four components: • one serving of fluid milk • one serving of M/MA • two servings of V/F • one serving of G/B	Increased quantities of V/F and G/B; otherwise, it is the same as the traditional approach	The number of menu items for the day must be offered in the planned quantities to meet the week's specified levels (with a minimum of three menu items): • fluid milk • entrée • side dish
Reimbursable lunch (*as served* standard)	• OVS is required in senior high schools[e]; students must select three of the five items • OVS is optional in grades below the senior high school level; schools may choose to have students select either three or four of the five items	Same as the traditional approach	OVS is required in senior high schools[e]; if three items are offered, students may decline one; if four or more items are offered, students may decline two • Students must always take the entrée • OVS is optional in grades below senior high school level • The number of menu items that students can decline is the same as stated above

Age-grade groups: Lunch	Established age-grade groups: • preschool • K–3 • grades 4–12 • grades 7–12 (optional)[f]	Established age-grade groups: preschool •K–6 •grades 7–12 •K–3 (optional)[f]	Options: • established grade groups: preschool, K–6 and 7–12 (K–3 optional)[f] • established age groups: ages 3–6, 7–10, 11–13, and 14–17; or • customized age groups
Reimbursable breakfast (*as offered* standard)[d]	A minimum of four required foods must be offered in specific quantities: • one serving of fluid milk, • one V/F, and • two M/MA or two G/B or one of each	Same as traditional approach	The number of menu items for the day must be offered in the planned quantities to meet the week's specified level (with a minimum of three menu items)
Reimbursable breakfast (*as served* standard) (OVS breakfast[g])	• Students must select at least three food items from the four items offered.	Same as traditional approach	• Students may decline a maximum of one menu item, regardless of the number of items offered
Age-grade groups: Breakfast	Established ages or grades: • preschool • K–12	Established ages or grades: •preschool •K–12 •grades 7–12 (optional)	Options: • established grade groups: preschool and K–12 (7–12 optional) • established age groups: ages 3–6, 7–10, 11–13, and 14 and older; or • customized age groups

NOTE: This table does not include information on the alternate menu planning approach (any reasonable approach). The state agency must approve any approach that differs in a major way from those listed in this table. G/B = grains and breads; K = kindergarten; M/MA = meat/meat alternate; OVS = offered versus served V/F = vegetables/fruits.

[a]Key elements of the Meal Requirements are designated by gray shading.

[b]See Appendix G for descriptions of the meal standards for the food components and food items.

[c]See Appendix H for descriptions of the meal standards for the nutrient-based menu planning approach.

[d]This is the standard that schools must meet when they are not operating under the OVS provisions.

[e]As defined by the state educational agency.

[f]Optional age-grade groups can be used if other established ages or groups do not accurately reflect the grades within that SFA.

[g]Offer versus serve is optional for all grades.

SOURCE: Adapted from USDA, 2007b.

NOTE: Excessive energy intakes for some age-gender groups may not have been identified because of underreporting.

Cost Reimbursement for Meals

Federal reimbursement of meal costs is the major source of cost reimbursement for meals and is conducted on the basis of prescribed record-keeping requirements, which are the responsibility of the SFA. Trained cashiers check the meals selected by the child against meal standards described in the previous section. Then, consistent with the level of reimbursement for that child, they tally the number of qualifying full-price, reduced-price, and free meals. This activity is shown at the end of the schematic in Figure 1-1 in Chapter 1. Meal reimbursement is intended for meals that have been prepared, offered, and selected consistent with the Nutrition Standards and Meal Requirements.

The three main budgetary inputs for providing high-quality, nutritious school meals that apply to both the NSLP and the SBP school meal programs are (1) federal per meal cash reimbursements, (2) the costs paid by participating children, and (3) the costs for USDA commodities. Two smaller federal programs also provide input. Each of these inputs is described briefly below.

Federal Cash Reimbursements

USDA provides per meal cash reimbursements to participating public and nonprofit private schools and residential child care institutions for meals that meet the federal Nutrition Standards. USDA provides the reimbursement to state agencies, which, in turn, disburse the monies to the SFAs within their states. In fiscal year (FY) 2007, cash payments were nearly $10 billion (USDA, 2008g).

The reimbursement rates for the 2008–2009 school year appear in Table 2-4. The reimbursement rate is adjusted annually on the basis of an index linked to the Consumer Price Index (which reflects changes in prices compared with those in the previous school year) and is published in the *Federal Register* by July 1 of each year to aid schools in planning for the new school year (*Amendments to the National School Lunch Act and the Child Nutrition Act,* P.L. 92-433, 1972).

TABLE 2-4 Federal per Meal Reimbursement Rates for School Meals in the Contiguous States, July 2008 Through June 2009

Program, Cost Basis[a]	Reimbursement Rates		
School breakfast	*Non-Severe Need*	*Severe Need*[b]	Cost of meal to child
Free	$1.40	$1.68	$0
Reduced price	$1.10	$1.38	≤$0.30
Paid	$0.25	$0.25	Varies[d]
School lunch	*<60% Were Free or Reduced Price*[c]	*≥60% Were Free or Reduced Price*[c]	
Free	$2.57	$2.59	$0
Reduced price	$2.17	$2.19	≤$0.40
Paid	$0.24	$0.26	Varies[d]

[a]Eligibility criteria are discussed in Chapter 1.
[b]Severe need refers to schools at which at least 60 percent of the lunches served during the second preceding school year were free or were provided at a reduced price (or, for new programs, if this requirement would have been met).
[c]Determined during the second preceding school year.
[d]Varies by school district or SFA.
SOURCE: USDA, 2008h.

Special provisions available through USDA (referred to as Provisions 1, 2, and 3) are aimed at reducing the application burden. The three provisions allow for providing meals at no cost to students, given that the schools follow certain application and claiming procedures (as outlined in regulation) (USDA, 2001c). Provision 1 is available to schools in which 80 percent of enrolled children are eligible for free or reduced-price meals. Students who qualify for free meals can be certified as eligible to receive them for a 2-year period. Provision 2 requires schools to provide free meals to all participating children and may certify children as eligible to receive free and reduced-price meals for up to a 4-year period. Provision 3 also requires schools to provide free meals to all participating children but changes the process by which federal cash and commodity assistance received by the school is determined (USDA, 2002c). The reimbursement rate for the free meals is the same as that indicated in Table 2-4.

Cost Paid by Participating Children

Meals are provided to children at either full price (called "paid" meals in Table 2-4), reduced-price, or free. By regulation, the cost of a meal to a child receiving a free or reduced-price meal may not be increased above the amount published in the *Federal Register* (currently the amount in the rightmost column of Table 2-4), but the cost for children paying full price may be set by the school district or SFA. Experience has shown that increasing the cost for full-price meals decreases the rate of participation by children living in households whose income exceeds the maximum allowed for reduced-price meals. In some cases, a decreased rate of participation may lead to higher per meal costs to the SFA because non-food costs do not decrease to the same degree. These limitations mean that the school food service planners must be very resourceful in controlling food, labor, and other costs, despite rising prices.

USDA Commodities

USDA agricultural commodities (called *commodities* here for convenience) are unprocessed or partially processed foods. USDA's Commodity Distribution Program began in response to the Depression in the 1930s. It assisted farmers by purchasing their surplus products, and it provided food for school lunches for millions of schoolchildren who were unable to pay for lunch (USDA, 2007c). The Commodity Distribution Program provides commodities to schools that participate in the NSLP. The overall value of the commodities provided was about $1 billion in FY 2007 (USDA, 2008g). The value of the commodities supplements the per meal cash reimbursements that schools receive. Local school districts are entitled to a specific dollar value of entitlement commodities each school year on the basis of the product of the total number of school lunches that they serve and a reimbursement rate. In addition, if USDA has a surplus of particular commodities, states may order whatever amount of these bonus commodities they can use. These do not count against a state's regular entitlement commodities. Market conditions and agricultural surpluses determine the availability of bonus commodities. In recent years, bonus commodities have become less common because of improved market conditions for agricultural producers, more precise crop planning, and tighter supply-chain management (CFPA, 2008).

State agencies may choose from a list of more than 180 different types of products, although they may decline offerings from the list if they choose not to include them in choices made available to the school districts. On the other hand, many states allow local school districts to choose from all available USDA commodity offerings. Foods that are available for the 2009 school year include fruits and vegetables, meats, dry and canned beans, fruit juices, vegetable shortening and vegetable oils, peanut products, rice, cheese, pasta products, and flour and other grain products (USDA, 2008i). Under the Processing Program that started in 1958, commercial food processors may contract with state agencies or school districts to convert raw bulk USDA commodities into products that are more convenient and ready to use (USDA, 2008j).

Much effort has been made to improve the available commodity offerings. Those offerings now include a larger proportion of fruits, vegetables, and whole grains, as well as products with reduced amounts of total fat, saturated fat, sugar, and sodium. *Trans* fats have been eliminated from frozen potato products and USDA is working to remove them from its other offerings (USDA, 2007d). Nonetheless, it can be a challenge for SFAs to fit the commodities into menus and recipes. Several federal agencies, the state distributing agency, and the school district are involved in decision making relating to the use of commodities on the basis of the choices of those districts.

Other Federal Programs That Provide Foods to Schools

Additionally, the U.S. Department of Defense Fresh Fruit and Vegetable Program operates a nationwide system that purchases and, in the 2006–2007 school year, distributed a wide variety of high-quality fresh produce to schools in 43 states, the District of Columbia, Puerto Rico, the Virgin Islands, and Guam (USDA, 2008k). The 2008 Farm Bill amended the National School Lunch Act to include the USDA Fresh Fruit and Vegetable Program. Beginning in the 2008–2009 school year, elementary schools could apply for funding to provide fresh fruits and vegetables to all students throughout the day if more than 50 percent of their student enrollment in the NSLP was comprised of students eligible for free and reduced-price meals (*Food, Conservation, and Energy Act of 2008,* P.L. 110-246 (June 18, 2008): § 4304).

TOPICS RELEVANT TO REVISING THE NUTRITION STANDARDS AND MEAL REQUIREMENTS

This section highlights a variety of topics that are relevant to the committee's task of recommending revisions to the Nutrition Standards and Meal Requirements. These include applying the *Dietary Guidelines for Americans* and the Dietary Reference Intakes (DRIs), addressing the need for simple approaches to making revisions, helping provide a safety net to children who are at risk of insufficient intake without contributing to excessive weight gain, planning meals that students will eat, addressing cost considerations, and addressing other factors that affect the feasibility of implementing the recommendations. Appendix E lists the critical issues included within the charge to the committee, most of which are mentioned in the discussions below.

Applying Dietary Guidelines to the School Meal Programs

Fruit, Vegetables, Whole Grains, and Low-Fat or Fat-Free Milk Products

The Child Nutrition and WIC Reauthorization Act of 2004 amended the National School Lunch Act to require the provision of increased amounts of foods that are recommended in the most recent *Dietary Guidelines for Americans*. These include fruits, vegetables, whole grains, and low-fat or fat-free milk products. The increased consumption of such food groups would likely call for the decreased consumption of other food groups (for example, meats and refined grains) and food components (such as hard fats or added sugars) or both to avoid excessive energy intake.

Addressing these issues requires the consideration of the FBMP and NBMP approaches. These two approaches and their meal standards currently differ with regard to the minimum number of servings and the minimum serving sizes of fruits and vegetables and fluid milk, and neither requires (but both encourage) the provision of whole grains. As shown in Table 2-3, the FBMP approaches are much more specific. The regulations specify that all schools must provide fluid milk in a variety of fat contents, but they do not restrict the types of fluid milk that are offered (*Child Nutrition and WIC Reauthorization Act,* P.L. 108-265 (June 30, 2004): § 102). The recommended daily intake of milk specified by the *Dietary Guidelines for Americans* is less for young children than for older children (see Appendix C), but offering smaller serving sizes to the younger children might lead to operational problems for SFAs that are working to provide meals to children who span a considerable age range.

The definition of whole grain will need to be considered. The method of assessing intake (see Chapter 4) distinguishes between 100 percent whole grain and various mixtures of grains. In the marketplace, most foods that contain whole grain have mixtures of grains. The term *whole grain* is not defined by Food and Drug Administration regulations, and the agency has not provided a definition of a whole-grain product or a whole-grain serving. To assess how well a school is meeting the Nutrition Standards should they include whole grains in menus, the definition of whole grain will need to be clear.

Sodium, Cholesterol, Fiber, and Trans Fat

The *Dietary Guidelines for Americans* include quantitative recommendations for limiting sodium and cholesterol intake and for increasing fiber intake. The guidelines also recommend limiting the intake of *trans* fat but do not specify an intake level. Especially with regard to limiting sodium intake, it may be challenging to obtain easily prepared foods that children will find appetizing.

Planning for Subsequent Revisions to Dietary Guidelines for Americans

By law, the need for revisions to the *Dietary Guidelines for Americans* must be addressed every 5 years. To date, the Dietary Guidelines Advisory Committees have recommended changes every 5 years. Especially since the next revision to *Dietary Guidelines for Americans* is expected in 2010, it may be helpful if the revisions for the Nutrition Standards and Meal Requirements for school meal programs can include a way to accommodate future changes to the *Dietary Guidelines for Americans.*

Applying Dietary Reference Intakes to the School Meal Programs

Relatively new nutrient reference values known as the DRIs (IOM, 1997, 1998, 2000a, 2001, 2002/2005, 2005) are now widely accepted and have even been incorporated into the *Dietary Guidelines for Americans*. The committee will examine ways to apply the DRIs to the development of revised Nutrition Standards for the school meal programs (The current Nutrition Standards are based on the 1989 RDAs.)

Incorporating the Dietary Reference Intake Planning Approaches for School Meals

A major element of the Institute of Medicine (IOM) report *Dietary Reference Intakes: Applications in Dietary Planning* (IOM, 2003) is the conclusion that the RDA is not an appropriate planning goal. Instead, the Estimated Average Requirement is the appropriate reference value to use to set a low prevalence of inadequacy as the planning goal. The IOM report provides some guidance on the planning of menus to achieve specified nutrient intakes and briefly addresses two options for the application of a framework for the planning of school meals for different age groups. The report also presents a nutrient density approach that may be applied to heterogeneous groups (groups that encompass individuals of both genders and individuals with different nutrient and energy requirements, which is the case in schools).

The report notes, however, that the planning task is complex and involves considerations related to program goals, nutritional aspects (such as the selection of target nutrient intake levels), and program implementation. It does not provide specific guidance on how to address the complexity of the task. The development of revisions to the Nutrition Standards and Meal Requirements for school meal programs must take the IOM planning report's guidance and related considerations into account.

Specifying Age-Grade Groups

Nutrient and energy needs differ by age and, in some cases, by gender. Currently, the regulations for school meal programs specify a number of age-grade groups (see Appendix G, for example) and make no distinction by gender. DRI age groups differ somewhat from the ages covered by the USDA-specified age-grade groups. The DRIs are set for children ages 4 through 8 years, 9 through 13 years, and 14 through 18 years; and they give separate values for males and females beginning at age 9 years.

Because of the discrepancies between the age-grade groups of the school meal programs and the age categories for DRIs, a range of nutrient values for a specific nutrient may apply to each age-grade group (see Chapter 5). During Phase II of this study, the committee will specify age-grade groups and propose the amounts of the required components of the Nutrition Standards by age-grade group (as was done in Table 2-2 for the current standards). These amounts would be used for nutrient-based menu planning and the evaluation of menus planned by use of the FBMP approach.

Recommending Energy Levels

Energy needs differ by age, as mentioned above, but also by physical activity level and body size (which vary greatly, especially in grades 7 through 12). Recommendations for energy will need to consider the great diversity of needs of the children being served. In the revision of Nutrition Standards and Meal Requirements, it may be appropriate to recommend both minimum and maximum energy levels.

Specifying Nutrients to Be Covered by the Nutrition Standards

Currently, regulations specify quantitative requirements for energy, protein, calcium, iron, vitamin A, vitamin C, total fat, and saturated fat (Table 2-1). In addition, the Nutrition Standards encourage program operators to reduce sodium and cholesterol levels and to increase fiber levels in the food items in their menus (the regulations provide no further specification). The DRIs include reference values for all of these nutrients plus many more, and the 2005 *Dietary Guidelines for Americans* (HHS/USDA, 2005) identified several nutrients of concern for children. These developments indicate the need for the reassessment of the nutrients covered in the Nutrition Standards.

Addressing the Need for Simple Approaches

Because revisions to the Nutrition Standards and Meal Requirements will need to be implemented in a wide variety of settings, one challenge is to develop standards whose implementation is simple enough for all food service operations, including those that face challenging operational problems or financial limitations.

School meals food service operations may differ in a variety of ways. These include but are not limited to the following:

- school size,
- number of schools served,
- number of children served,
- the grades of the children served,
- the distance of the feeding site from the kitchen,
- funding,
- the qualifications and training of the food service personnel,
- the computer expertise of the SFA,
- the number of personnel relative to the task,
- the menu planning approach used,
- the time available to serve meals,
- equipment and storage facilities, and
- the cultural and socioeconomic diversity of the student body.

Evidence suggests that the implementation of the approaches and standards put forth by the SMI has required careful planning, resources, and time. To facilitate the implementation of the Nutrition Standards and the serving of appropriate meals, USDA has made many resources available to school food service operators. For example, USDA provides a computer disk called *SMI Tools for Success for School Food Authorities* that contains a 71-page document called *SMI Frequently Asked Questions*, a 125-page document called *The Road to SMI Success*, and a 127-page document called *Nutrient Analysis Protocols: How to Analyze Menus for USDA's School Meals Programs*. USDA offers grants for training program operators on SMI guidelines to state agencies as well. Nonetheless, the implementation of SMI has been challenging for many SFAs, as indicated in Chapter 1.

Providing a Safety Net for Vulnerable Children Without Contributing to Excessive Weight Gain

From their inception, the school meal programs have played a key role in providing a safety net for low-income U.S. children to help ensure that they are well fed. As obesity has become a common occurrence among the nation's children, however, many people are concerned that revisions to Nutrition Standards and Meal Requirements for school meals consider both the potential contributions of school meals to childhood obesity and to fostering the food security of children, where food security[5] means "access at all times to enough food for an active, healthy life" (IOM, 2006a).

Low Food Security

Low food security is described as "reports of reduced quality, variety, or desirability of the diet" and "little or no indication of reduced food intake" (USDA/ERS, 2007a, table) in the household. *Very low food security* is described as "reports of multiple indications of disrupted eating patterns and reduced food intake" in the household (USDA/ERS, 2007a, table). The prevalence of low food security varies inversely with changing economic conditions; the prevalence increases when economic conditions worsen. Between 1995 and 2005, 14.8 to 17.6 percent of U.S. households with children under the age of 18 years were assessed to be food insecure. For logistical reasons, these data exclude approximately 800,000 to 1.2 million homeless children (NCH, 2008), who are likely to be at high risk of disrupted eating patterns and reduced food intake. Overall, 0.8 percent of children lived in a household with very low food security, in which limited food availability was reported to have led to restricted intake for one or more children in the household (USDA/ERS, 2006).

Relationships of Low Food Security with Body Weight Status

In the United States, low food security does not appear to be associated with underweight in schoolchildren (Bhattacharya et al., 2004). In fact, less than 3 percent of children ages 5 through 18 years were classified as underweight in an analysis of the data from the 1999–2004 National Health and Nutrition Examination Survey (USDA, 2008l). Importantly, it appears that children in households with low food security are as likely or more likely to be obese or overweight than children in food-secure households (Alaimo et al., 2001; Bhattacharya et al., 2004; Casey et al., 2006; Martin and Ferris, 2007; Gunderson et al., 2008). In a recent study of children ages 10

[5]Hunger and food security are global issues, and related definitions used in other countries vary.

through 15 years, Gunderson et al. (2008) reported that 25 percent of the children in households with low food security had body mass indexes that were greater than the 95th percentile of Centers for Disease Control and Prevention growth charts (obese). About one-third of all schoolchildren are overweight or obese (Table 1-2 in Chapter 1). The revision of the Nutrition Standards and Meal Requirements will need to help ensure that school meals contribute to both food security and healthy weight.

Planning Meals That Students Will Eat

Revisions to the Nutrition Standards and Meal Requirements will be valuable only to the extent that students consume the food that is served. Reportedly, a major hurdle to the potential revisions is a lack of student acceptance of the changes brought about by the revisions (SNA/SNF, 2007). One study reported that the significant factors affecting students' decisions to participate in the NSLP were the quality and the variety of foods offered (Marples and Spillman, 1995). Wojcicki and Heyman (2006) found that the availability of healthy food options on the menu was followed by higher rates of student participation in the NSLP. Other factors, however, may have been related to the increase in participation, such as increased eligibility for free and reduced-price meals. Some schools provide self-service salad bars to encourage the consumption of greater amounts of fruits and vegetables. Nevertheless, Adams et al. (2005) found no association between the availability of salad bars and fruit and vegetable consumption, but they did find that the consumption of fruits and vegetables was positively related to the number of those items offered at the salad bars.

Certain types of menu changes offered to improve the rates of adherence to the *Dietary Guidelines for Americans* could have an adverse effect on student acceptability of school meals and, therefore, on the rate of program participation, especially if the changes are made in an abrupt manner. On the other hand, Wechslar and colleagues (1998) reported that the implementation of strategies to promote the acceptance of low-fat milk in elementary schools in an inner-city neighborhood doubled its selection (to 57 percent of the milk selected). Such factors will need to be considered during the process of updating the standards.

Based on information available, meal acceptance is a factor to be taken into account in making recommendations to update the Nutrition Standards and Meal Requirements. However, as a general matter, student acceptance of foods is a complex topic for which there are relatively little data and many unknowns. To appropriately address the issue in a way that provides pragmatic guidance for practitioners requires considerations outside the scope of this study. Relevant topics may range from the discovery that children drink milk more readily if it is packaged in a carton showing a favorite cartoon character, to experimenting with recipes that are low in sodium but use spices acceptable to children to "up" the flavor. Such information is important for implementation of new meal standards, but much of the research is only now emerging.

Addressing Cost Considerations

Many factors affect the cost of school meal programs. Among these factors are the costs of food, labor, utilities, and fuel (for off-site delivery); indirect costs; equipment depreciation; and the availability of federal commodities to the program. Some of these factors are influenced by the number of children served, by changes in the operation of public schools (e.g., subdividing large high schools into smaller free-standing units), the number of children with special health care needs that include dietary modifications, state and local purchasing options, and the cultural diversity of the school population.

In difficult economic times, an increasing number of school food service operations are required to cover all their costs without receiving financial support from the school district. In many parts of the country, there is debate about whether school meal programs should be self-supporting or whether they should be subsidized to some degree because the provision of nutritious meals is part of the mission of the school.

Importantly for this study, it has been found that the improved implementation of current Nutrition Standards typically results in increased costs at the local level. In a survey conducted to examine the implementation of school wellness policies, 78 percent of school districts reported increased costs, mainly as a result of the increased cost of food (SNA/SNF, 2007). Further improvements in menus may contribute to further cost increases. Therefore, revisions to the Nutrition Standards and Meal Requirements will need to consider costs. As USDA does not anticipate that additional funding will be available to schools so that they may implement any new revisions of the Nutrition Standards and Meal Requirements resulting from the committee's recommendations, the request to the committee is that recommendations be designed to be economical.

Other Factors Affecting Feasibility

The feasibility of implementing recommendations for revisions to the Nutrition Standards and related Meal Requirements may be affected by the factors mentioned above that relate to the complexity or the simplicity of the recommendations, the diversity of food service operations and facilities, personnel, cost, student acceptability, and student participation. Among the other factors that may affect the feasibility of implementing the revisions are the following:

- *Variability in the methods that states and districts use to operate the school meal programs.* Federal regulations set minimum requirements for Nutrition Standards and Meal Requirements for the operation of school meal programs; but states may add requirements, and many do so.
- *Determining the contribution of mixed foods to meeting the meal standards.* The food group contributions of the components of purchased products such as pizza, beef patties (which differ in their fat contents), and certain juice products (which differ in the percentage of juice) can be difficult to determine. The USDA's Food and Nutrition Service works directly with commercial food-processing firms and operates a voluntary federal labeling program called the Child Nutrition (CN) Labeling Program. Figure 2-2 shows an example of a CN label. Costs are associated with obtaining the approved CN label.

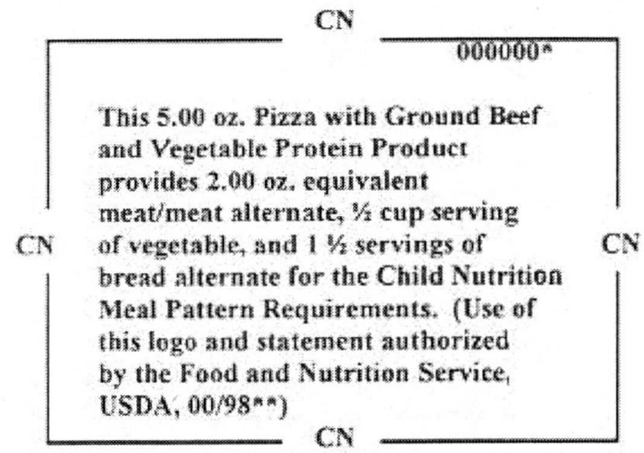

FIGURE 2-2 Example of a CN label. A CN label specifies the number of portions of one or more food groups that one serving of the food provides.
SOURCE: USDA, 2008m.

- *Available nutrient information.* By law (*Nutrition Labeling and Education Act of 1990*, P.L. 101-535), the current Nutrition Facts panel on food labels includes information on the product's content of the 11 nutrients listed in Table 2-1. The law does not require the listing of any other nutrients. Some of the nutrients that were identified in the *Dietary Guidelines for Americans* as nutrients of concern for children (such as potassium, magnesium, and vitamin E) are listed on few food labels (manufacturers may list these and other nutrients at their discretion). Products that bear the CN label are not required to have a Nutrition Facts panel; however some manufacturers add the panel to CN-labeled products voluntarily. Since SMI reviews require that nutrition information for all commercially prepared food products is kept on file, SFAs can contact the manufacturer directly to obtain that information. Because many school meal program operators rely on information obtained from food labels and product specifications to plan and assess menus, the availability of nutrient information merits consideration.
- *Expression of the vitamin A standard.* If proposed revisions include a standard for vitamin A intake, consideration will need to be given to the difference in units used in the DRIs (Retinol Activity Equivalents) and on the Nutrition Facts panel and product specifications (international units). The availability of a method for conversion from one to the other set of units would be useful. Currently, only schools using the NBMP and USDA-approved software are able to calculate and report the nutrient analysis in both units (USDA, 2006a).
- *Flexibility of the SBP and menu structures.* Current regulations provide schools with the flexibility to provide a typical breakfast that minimizes the burden on school food service operations and encourages broad participation in the SBP. Consideration may need to be given to maintaining such flexibility while improving compliance with the *Dietary Guidelines for Americans*.
- *Portion sizes.* Offering different portion sizes (especially of prepackaged foods, such as fluid milk) to accommodate the different nutritional needs of children in different grades may be operationally difficult to implement at the local school level. Attention to procurement logistics and economies of scale that may pose limitations to this approach is warranted.
- *The school nutrition and health environment.* The increased consumption of foods from the school meal programs rather than of competitive foods has been shown to improve dietary intake (Cullen et al., 2008). Nevertheless, in many schools, reimbursable meals have competition from foods that are available à la carte and at snack bars, school stores, canteens, and vending

machines. In many cases, these options have been introduced with the intent of generating income to benefit the school or to help the school food operation break even. Indeed, according to the School Health Profiles survey (CDC, 2008b), a large majority of secondary schools in 27 states and 11 large urban school districts allowed students to buy competitive foods onsite. Thus, for schools that retain these options, reimbursable meals planned to meet revised Nutrition Standards and Meal Requirements need to be sufficiently attractive to students so that students chose the school meals rather than the other options. Factors found to affect students' decision to participate in the school lunch program include the length of the lunch period and the amount of time that one must stand in line to obtain the food (Marples and Spillman, 1995). Thus, meal patterns that lend themselves to quick service may be beneficial. The report *Nutrition Standards for Foods in Schools* (IOM, 2007) addresses in detail the school environment and the foods and beverages sold outside the school meal programs.

- *The market environment.* Some of the challenges in revising the Nutrition Standards and Meal Requirements for school meals extend beyond the efforts of program operators and administrators. For example, many of the processed foods that are used in school meal programs to save time and reduce labor costs are high in sodium. If revised standards call for foods that differ from those offered in the general market, the food industry would require time to respond with palatable products.

SUMMARY

As described in this chapter, the revision of the Nutrition Standards and Meal Requirements for the school meal programs necessitates attention to a large number of topics. These topics range from updates in dietary and nutrient recommendations to the feasibility of implementing the changes and the costs involved. The next chapter describes the committee's working principles, criteria, and overall approach to developing recommendations for revisions to the NSLP and the SBP.

3

Working Principles and Criteria for the Committee's Approach to Proposing Revisions

The members of the Committee on Nutrition Standards for National School Lunch and Breakfast Programs developed working principles and criteria to assist them with developing recommendations for revisions to the Nutrition Standards and Meal Requirements of the school meal programs. The working principles are intended to guide committee deliberations, and the proposed set of criteria will be applied during the development of the committee's recommendations for revision. This chapter presents these principles, the proposed criteria, and an overview of the proposed approach to developing recommendations for revisions.

WORKING PRINCIPLES

The working principles shown in Box 3-1 take into account the committee's task (stated in Chapter 1), an array of background information on the need for the revisions (summarized in Chapter 1), topics relevant to revising the standards (summarized in Chapter 2), and the critical areas for consideration listed in Appendix E.

BOX 3-1
Working Principles for Determining Recommendations for Revisions to the Nutrition Standards and Meal Requirements for School Meals

1. The present and future health and well-being of schoolchildren are profoundly affected by their food and nutrient intakes and the maintenance of healthy body weight.
    a. School meals, when they are consumed, should improve food and nutrient intakes, and those intakes that are inadequate or excessive in school-age children should specifically be targeted.
    b. School meals are targeted to children ages 4 through 17 years, but younger children and children of all ages with special needs may be affected by the standards set for the general population.
    c. Recognition will be given to health effects of foods (including beverages) that go beyond those related to their nutrient content.
2. School lunch and breakfast programs, which may contribute to more than 50 percent of the caloric intake by children on school days, offer opportunities to promote the health and well-being of children.
    a. School meals can contribute to beneficial health and dietary patterns and are uniquely positioned to provide a model for healthy meals and to provide opportunities to model and reinforce healthy eating behaviors.
    b. School meals can provide a platform for education in nutrition, environmental responsibility, and food safety.
    c. School meals can be a positive environment for pleasant social interactions.
    d. For children in families characterized by limited resources and food insecurity, school meals provide a critical safety net in meeting their nutritional needs and reducing the adverse effects of food insecurity.
3. School lunch and breakfast programs operate in a challenging and changing environment.
    a. School food service environments (such as facilities, equipment, labor, and skills) are complex and highly varied across the nation as well as from school to school within school districts.
    b. Challenges include the need to meet food safety standards, offer appetizing foods to an increasingly diverse population, adjust to the changes in the available food supply, improve the image and appeal of the program, and achieve a sound financial operation.
    c. Food costs, other direct costs, and indirect costs related to program operation are outpacing the available resources.
    d. In addition to promoting the health and well-being of children, high rates of participation may support the financial stability of school meal programs.
    e. Efforts to change the current school nutrition environments vary, with some districts already making significant strides and others just starting the process of change.
4. Because scientific findings and authoritative recommendations related to the nutrition of children evolve over time, the process of developing recommendations for revisions should be transparent and designed to take into account new evidence-based findings and recommendations.

CRITERIA

On the basis of the evidence considered during its Phase I activities, the committee proposes four criteria that can be used to derive and evaluate the recommendations that will be made during Phase II of the study. The criteria are identified and discussed below.

CRITERION 1

THE NUTRITION STANDARDS AND MEAL REQUIREMENTS WILL BE CONSISTENT WITH CURRENT DIETARY GUIDANCE AND NUTRITION RECOMMENDATIONS TO PROMOTE HEALTH—AS EXEMPLIFIED BY THE *DIETARY GUIDELINES FOR AMERICANS* AND THE DIETARY REFERENCE INTAKES—WITH THE ULTIMATE GOAL OF IMPROVING CHILDREN'S DIETS BY REDUCING THE APPARENT PREVALENCE OF INADEQUATE AND EXCESSIVE INTAKES OF FOOD, NUTRIENTS, AND CALORIES.

MyPyramid, which is based on the 2005 *Dietary Guidelines for Americans* (HHS/USDA, 2005), provides concrete recommendations for food intakes; and the Dietary Reference Intakes provide reference values for nutrient intakes. However, because school meals are provided to groups of children with a range of ages, body sizes, and activity levels, the committee cannot apply the values and recommendations directly to the Nutrition Standards and Meal Requirements. In deriving the recommendations, the committee will give special attention to the following aspects of providing healthful amounts of food groups, food subgroups, and nutrients, as requested by USDA:

- appropriate levels of total fat, saturated fat, cholesterol, and *trans* fat in school meals;
- the inclusion of specific foods whose consumptions should be encouraged on the basis of the recommendations of the *Dietary Guidelines for Americans*, that is, fruit, vegetables, whole grains, and nonfat or low-fat milk products;
- provisions for healthful levels of sodium and fiber;
- nutrients and other dietary components of concern, as identified in the assessment of intakes by schoolchildren; and
- calorie levels provided at lunch and breakfast that are sufficient to meet the child's energy needs at those meals but that do not promote excessive energy intake.

To help reduce the possibility of excessive energy intake, maximum calorie levels for school meals will be considered. Criterion 1 refers to the "apparent prevalence of inadequate and excessive intakes" because adequacy, inadequacy, and excessive intake cannot be determined from dietary assessment alone. Throughout this report, terms such as "adequate intake," "excessive intake," and "nutrient intake" are used. The reader should recognize that phrases such as "apparently adequate intake" and "apparent nutrient inadequacy" would be more precise. We have omitted the qualifier for ease of reading.

If some of the nutrients or other dietary components of concern differ from the nutrients whose amounts are required to be listed on food labels, in accordance with the provisions of the Nutrition Labeling and Education Act (P.L. 101-535, 1990), the committee will consider the most effective ways to address labeling for these nutrients in implementing the recommendations for revisions to Nutrient Standards and Meal Requirements.

CRITERION 2

THE NUTRITION STANDARDS AND MEAL REQUIREMENTS WILL BE CONSIDERED ON THE BASIS OF AGE-GRADE GROUPS THAT ARE CONSISTENT WITH THE CURRENT AGE-GENDER CATEGORIES USED FOR SPECIFYING REFERENCE VALUES AND WITH WIDELY USED SCHOOL GRADE CONFIGURATIONS.

The committee will continue its deliberations and analyses related to the current common configurations for school grade categories and make recommendations for revisions to the Nutrition Standards and Meal Requirements for the appropriate age-grade groups.

CRITERION 3

THE NUTRITION STANDARDS AND MEAL REQUIREMENTS WILL RESULT IN THE SIMPLIFICATION OF THE MENU PLANNING AND MONITORING PROCESSES, AND THEY WILL BE COMPATIBLE WITH THE DEVELOPMENT OF MENUS THAT ARE PRACTICAL TO PREPARE AND SERVE AND THAT OFFER NUTRITIOUS FOODS AND BEVERAGES THAT APPEAL TO STUDENTS.

The committee recognizes that increasing complexity of program operations and related standards may challenge the success of the programs. The limited resources to both train and manage staff means that the school lunch and breakfast programs will operate best if the requirements and standards are practical and as straightforward as possible. Further, the committee's intent is to propose revisions that will encourage wide participation in the school meal programs. Included among the key factors that affect menu appeal and acceptability by students are sodium content, the availability of choices, and familiarity with the food on the basis of the student's cultural background or previous experience consuming the food (such as nonfat or low-fat milk). The committee will give consideration to the *as served* option in this regard and also to any relevant plate-waste studies. Furthermore, the committee recognizes the challenges that may occur pertaining to student acceptance of meals planned in line with the recommendations—for example, if the menu items offered contain less sodium and saturated fat and more fiber and whole grains. As feasible within the scope of work of this study, the committee will consider these challenges as it develops recommendations for the Nutrition Standards and Meal Requirements.

The committee will develop a sample 4-week cycle of menus to ensure that it is possible to meet the nutrient- and food-related recommendations, but also to examine and illustrate the practicality and flexibility of implementation of the Nutrition Standards and Meal Requirements. School districts are ultimately responsible for developing menus and selecting food items that appeal to their students, so practicality and flexibility of implementation are essential. Meal standards apply to diverse school food authorities with widely different physical production plants and other resources. One essential element will be the availability of palatable food products with appropriate nutrient profiles that are in forms that can easily be incorporated into school meals. The committee will also consider the ability to simplify the menu-planning approaches available to school food authorities.

CRITERION 4

THE NUTRITION STANDARDS AND MEAL REQUIREMENTS WILL BE SENSITIVE TO PROGRAM COSTS.

Because certain improvements to the Nutrition Standards and Meal Requirements have the potential to increase food costs or other direct or indirect costs of school meals, or both, the committee will explore ways to control program costs.

OVERVIEW OF THE COMMITTEE'S PROPOSED APPROACH TO DEVELOPING RECOMMENDATIONS

The committee's proposed approach to developing recommendations for revisions to the Nutrition Standards and Meal Requirements for the National School Lunch Program (NSLP) and the School Breakfast Program (SBP) includes the following four steps:

1. applying the working principles to guide the selection of data and the types of analyses and reviews to be conducted and to focus committee deliberations;
2. assessing the dietary intakes of food groups, food subgroups, and nutrients by schoolchildren to identify the food and nutrient intakes of concern for selected age groups;
3. examining various approaches to planning the nutritional aspects of school meals so that the recommendations for revisions to the Nutrition Standards and the Meal Requirements may be effectively incorporated into the requirements for the meals. The committee plans to use iterative processes to derive the recommendations that best meet all five criteria; and
4. applying the criteria listed above in the development of the committee's recommendations for revisions to the Nutrition Standards and Meal Requirements. This will include
    a. incorporating sensitivity analysis to examine the nutritional impacts of the recommended revisions, and
    b. addressing the cost implications and market effects of the recommended revisions.

An initial assessment of food and nutrient needs appears in Chapter 4. The development of a proposed planning model that may be used to develop recommendations for revisions to the NSLP and the SBP is discussed in Chapter 5. Finally, Chapter 6 presents proposals for incorporating the findings of the sensitivity analysis and for addressing cost implications and market effects.

4

Food and Nutrient Needs of Schoolchildren

The committee's charge included a requirement to "review and assess the food and nutritional needs of school-aged children in the United States based on the 2005 Dietary Guidelines and the Dietary Reference Intakes." Findings from this review are to form the basis for recommended revisions to existing nutrition standards and meal requirements. In its review, the committee considered recent published data on schoolchildren in the United States covering the children's dietary intakes, weight status, and biochemical indicators of nutritional status. This chapter describes the data used in the committee's review, including details about the methods for assessing the apparent adequacy of children's food and nutrient intakes. Then it summarizes the committee's key findings in two sections. The first section addresses the children's reported food intakes, and the second addresses children's estimated energy and nutrient intakes. The chapter concludes with the identification of food groups and nutrients under consideration for special attentions during Phase II of the study.

DATA SOURCES

The data considered by the committee came primarily from two published studies that included nationally representative samples of schoolchildren in the United States:

- ***Diet Quality of American School-Age Children by School Lunch Participation Status* (USDA, 2008l).** This report, hereafter referred to as the 2008 Diet Quality Report, used data from the National Health and Nutrition Examination Survey (NHANES). NHANES is conducted by the National Center for Health Statistics and is designed to provide national estimates of the health and nutrition status of the civilian, noninstitutionalized population in the 50 states. Since 1999, NHANES has been a continuous annual survey, and data from the survey are released in public data files every 2 years. The 2008 Diet Quality Report provides data on children's 1-day (24-hour) intakes of MyPyramid food groups (USDA, 2008n), on the basis of data from

NHANES 1999–2002,[1] and on children's usual nutrient intakes[2] and body weight distributions, on the basis of data from NHANES 1999–2004.

- ***School Nutrition Dietary Assessment Study–III* (SNDA-III) (USDA, 2007a).** SNDA-III was sponsored by the U.S. Department of Agriculture (USDA) and collected data from a nationally representative sample of public school children in grades 1–12. The study's multistage sampling approach first sampled school food authorities (SFAs) in the 48 contiguous states, then the schools served by those SFAs, and then the children who attended those schools. SNDA-III provides data on children's usual nutrient intakes. Data were collected during the 2004–2005 school year.

Table 4-1 summarizes information about each of these main data sources and how they were used in the committee's review. Additional details about the data collection methods, the samples analyzed, and the analysis methods are provided in Appendix I. Neither of the two main data sources included information about *trans* fat or vitamin D intakes, but the committee briefly addressed these two topics in its review. To supplement the available data, the committee reviewed published reports of NHANES data on (1) body mass index and the prevalence of obesity, and (2) biochemical indicators of nutritional status.

TABLE 4-1 Key Data Sources Used to Assess Food and Nutrient Needs of Schoolchildren

	2008 Diet Quality Report[a]	SNDA-III[b]
Data reviewed by the Committee		
One-day food group intakes based on MyPyramid*	√	—
Usual nutrient intakes	√	√
BMI Distribution	√	—
Sample	• Children (ages 5–18 years) • One-day intakes of MyPyramid food groups: 2,597 children • Usual nutrient intakes: 3,546 children • BMI distribution: 3,495 children	2,314 children (ages 6–18 years)
Data collection period	• One-day intakes of MyPyramid food groups: 1999–2002 • Usual nutrient intakes and BMI distribution: 1999–2004	2004–2005 school year

NOTE: — = data not included; √ = data included; SNDA=School Nutrition Dietary Assessment.

*Data on food group intakes were based on a single 24-hour recall and were not adjusted to reflect usual food intakes. Analysis was limited appropriately to estimates of group means.

SOURCES: [a] USDA, 2008l; [b] USDA, 2007a.

[1]MyPyramid intakes could not be estimated for children in the NHANES 2002–2004 sample because a companion database that is needed to generate these estimates (the MyPyramid Equivalents Database for USDA Food Codes [version 1.0; USDA, 2006b]), provides data only for NHANES 1999–2000 and 2001–2002.

[2]"Usual nutrient intakes" refers to 24-hour recall data that have been statistically adjusted, following methods recommended by the IOM, to better estimate long-run (usual) intakes (ISU, 1997; Nusser et al., 1996); for this report, reference to nutrient intake includes energy (calories).

DATA LIMITATIONS

Dietary intake data played a central role in the committee's review and assessment of children's food and nutrient needs, as shown in Table 4-1. The available data have four important limitations that the committee acknowledged in its review. Each of these limitations is described below.

Underreporting and Overreporting of Food Intakes

It is well recognized that individuals responding to dietary surveys may underreport or overreport their intakes. Underreporting may result in overestimates of the prevalence of inadequate intakes or in underestimates of excessive intakes; and overreporting may result in overestimates of excessive intakes (Briefel et al., 1997). Underreporting tends to be greatest among adolescents, especially females; people who are overweight or obese; and people who have low incomes (Bandini et al., 1997; Braam et al., 1998; Little et al., 1999; Livingstone et al., 1992; Pryer et al., 1997; Stallone et al., 1997; Ventura et al., 2006). For elementary school-age children, the opposite problem may occur, with food intakes being overreported by the children themselves, by their parents, or by both (Basch et al., 1990; Baxter et al., 2002; Lytle et al., 1993). Some researchers have reported that there may be differences in children's under- and overreporting by meal (Baxter et al., 2007; Guinn et al., 2008).

Problems of underreporting in the data reviewed by the committee may have been mitigated to some extent by the data collection processing techniques used:

- Both NHANES and SNDA-III used the Automated Multiple-Pass Method (AMPM) which limits the underreporting of food intakes (Johnson et al., 2008) and improves the accuracy of estimated energy intakes in normal weight adults (Moshfegh et al., 2008).
- SNDA-III used several data collection strategies to minimize reporting errors among children (USDA, 2007a) that included two-part interviewing and parental assistance for elementary school children, aids for the interviews such as copies of school menus, and a listing of all potential locations in a school where food or beverages could be obtained.
- SNDA-III incorporated data provided by school foodservice managers about portion sizes used and energy and nutrient content of foods offered in reimbursable school meals before processing the 24-hour recall data.

Although the above techniques may have acted to reduce reporting errors in the NHANES and SNDA-III dietary intake data, there is evidence to suggest that some level of under- or overreporting remains. Moshfegh et al. (2008) found that, even with use of the AMPM protocol, individuals who were overweight or obese underreported their energy intakes. Moreover, as discussed later in this chapter, the SNDA-III data provide suggestive evidence that the intakes of children ages 6–8 years and females ages 9–13 years may have been overreported and that intakes of adolescents ages 14–18 years, particularly males, may have been underreported. It is likely that comparable over- and underreporting occurred in the NHANES data used in the 2008 Diet Quality Report; however the committee did not have access to data that would elucidate this issue.[3] The major implications of the apparent over- and underreporting of food intakes is that

---

[3]The SNDA-III report included comparisons of reported energy intakes and Estimated Energy Requirements (EERs). These comparisons suggest come misreporting of usual food (energy) intakes. Because the 2008 Diet

the prevalence of nutrient inadequacy may be underestimated for children ages 6–8 years and for females ages 9–13 years, but it may be overestimated for adolescents ages 14–18 years.

Despite these limitations, the dietary intake data are an important source of information for the committee's work. The method recommended by the Institute of Medicine (IOM, 2000b) to assess the adequacy of diets consumed by population groups requires the use of 24-hour recall data. The committee agrees with the Institute of Medicine that "comparing high-quality intake data with tailored requirement data to assess intakes is a meaningful undertaking and can, at a minimum, identify nutrients likely to be either under- or overconsumed by the … group of interest" (IOM, 2000b, p. 161). The committee recognizes that estimates of the prevalence of inadequate nutrient intakes are imprecise, providing general information about nutrients that are most likely to be of concern rather than precise estimates of the proportions of children with definitive nutrient inadequacies. The committee also examined anthropometric data and biochemical data to obtain additional perspective on children's usual intakes of energy and micronutrients, respectively.

One-Day Data on Food Group Intakes Rather Than Usual Intakes

The available data on children's food group intakes are based on a single 24-hour recall, whereas data on nutrient intakes reflect children's usual intakes. Although data from a single 24-hour recall do not provide a reliable estimate of an individual's usual intake or the usual intake distribution of a population group, these data do provide reliable estimates of mean intakes at the group level. Consequently, the committee's use of the food intake data is limited to examination of mean intakes relative to MyPyramid recommendations.

Lack of Data on Supplement Intake

Nutrient intakes from both the 2008 Diet Quality Report and SNDA-III are based on intakes from food and beverages only. They do not include intakes from dietary supplements or over-the-counter medicines. The 2008 Diet Quality Report indicated that 29 percent of all schoolchildren took some type of dietary supplement (most commonly multivitamin-multimineral preparations) during the preceding month, and SNDA-III found that more than half of all schoolchildren used vitamin supplements at some level. Given that sizeable proportions of schoolchildren used supplements, nutrient intake data from both SNDA-III and the 2008 Diet Quality Report may overestimate the prevalence of nutrient inadequacy. In addition, it was generally not possible to determine whether nutrients were consumed in amounts that were higher than the Tolerable Upper Intake Level (UL).

Lag in Reflecting Changes in the Marketplace

Recent changes in food fortification and in other aspects of the marketplace may have changed the availability and the consumption of some types of food and some nutrients and other food components. For example, the availability of whole grain products and of calcium-fortified foods has been increasing, and the *trans* fat content of foods has been decreasing. However, the impacts of marketplace changes on consumption among schoolchildren is unknown.

Quality Report did not include comparisons of usual energy intakes and EERs, it was not possible to assess the likelihood of over- or underreporting.

ASSESSMENT OF FOOD INTAKES

To assess children's food intakes, the committee relied on data from the 2008 Diet Quality Report. These data are based on single 24-hour recalls collected in NHANES 1999–2002. The MyPyramid food guidance system (USDA, 2008n) provided the recommended levels of intake that the committee used to assess food intakes (see Appendix J). The committee used the MyPyramid food guidance system because it translates the 2005 *Dietary Guidelines for Americans* (HHS/USDA, 2005) into recommendations about the types and amounts of food that should be consumed to promote health and maintain weight (Marcoe et al., 2006).

The MyPyramid Food Guidance System

The MyPyramid food guidance system (USDA, 2008n) includes MyPyramid food intake patterns. These patterns provide specific food-based dietary guidance that is consistent with the recommendations in the 2005 *Dietary Guidelines for Americans*. The system also incorporates the nutrient-based recommendations made in the Dietary Reference Intakes (DRIs). USDA used an iterative process to develop the food intake patterns for MyPyramid. This process identified appropriate energy levels and nutritional goals for the patterns, established food groupings, determined the amounts of nutrients that would be provided by consuming different combinations of foods, and evaluated the nutrient levels in each pattern against specific goals. With the exception of sodium, nutrient goals were set by using the Recommended Dietary Allowances (RDAs) or Adequate Intakes (AIs). For sodium, the goal was less than the UL. USDA used a weighted average to estimate the amounts of nutrients that each food group would contribute. The assigned weights were based on the level of consumption of each food item, as determined from national food consumption surveys (Marcoe et al., 2006).

Appendix J presents tables from MyPyramid that provide the food intake patterns (recommended types and amounts of foods) for various calorie levels suitable for schoolchildren. The MyPyramid food intake patterns provide at least 90 percent of the goals for all nutrients except vitamin E and potassium. The amounts of vitamin E and potassium provided by the patterns are larger, however, than the typical intakes by children (Marcoe et al., 2006).

The major food groups in MyPyramid are fruits, vegetables, grains, milk products, meat and meat alternates, and oils.[4] To promote the intake of the recommended amounts of nutrients, food intake patterns specify five subgroups for vegetables (dark green vegetables, orange vegetables, legumes, starchy vegetables, and other vegetables) and two subgroups for grains (whole grains and other grains).

The foods used to develop the food patterns are the forms of each food in the food group that are the lowest in fat (e.g., lean meat and fat-free milk) and that are free of added sugars (e.g., water-packed canned fruit). Thus, the patterns assume the consumption of the most nutrient-dense forms of foods in each food group. The MyPyramid food guide also includes a discretionary calorie allowance, that is, the amount of calories from any source (often added sugars or solid fats) that can be used flexibly. For the purposes of this Phase I report and its related analyses, considerations concerning added sugars are included as a component of the discretionary calorie allowance. During Phase II, issues related to added sugars in school meal programs will be considered more specifically.

---

[4]Oils and *trans*-free soft margarines are included to provide vitamin E and essential fatty acids.

Table J-2 in Appendix J provides detailed information about the food items included in each food group and subgroup[5]; the equivalent quantities for each food group; and explanations of the recommended amounts for the vegetable and grain subgroups, oils, and the discretionary calorie allowance. The explanations are key to understanding new concepts that were introduced on the basis of the work of the 2005 Dietary Guidelines Advisory Committee (HHS/USDA, 2004).

MyPyramid includes food intake patterns for a wide range of calorie levels to accommodate the needs of different individuals. (Appendix J shows only the intake patterns that are suitable for children ages 2–18 years.) The recommended amounts of foods from the major food groups and from the food subgroups differ with differences in nutrient and energy needs, which are based on a person's age, gender, and activity level. Mean food group intakes that are below MyPyramid recommendations do not necessarily indicate inadequate nutrient intake, but they do suggest improvements to the diet that would achieve greater consistency with *Dietary Guidelines for Americans* and recommended intakes for individuals.

Estimating Intakes of MyPyramid Food Groups

The committee relied on published estimates of children's one day intakes of MyPyramid food groups. Estimation of the intakes of MyPyramid food groups is a complex process for several reasons: (1) a large percentage of the foods eaten in the United States represent a combination of ingredients from two or more food groups, (2) many of the foods consumed are not lean or fat-free forms of the food, and (3) many foods contain added solid fats or added sugars, or both.

Cleveland and colleagues (1997) developed a method that can be used to analyze food intake data to estimate the number of Food Pyramid servings for comparison with Pyramid recommendations. (The Food Pyramid was an earlier version of the MyPyramid food guidance system.) The method involves the disaggregation of food mixtures into their component parts so that each ingredient can be credited to a specific food group. For example, the ingredients in pizza are credited to the grains, milk, vegetable, and (if meat is present) the meat and meat alternates groups.[6] If the meat is not lean, the number of grams of fat in excess of a lean meat ounce equivalent would be considered discretionary calories. The grain in a sweetened ready-to-eat cereal would be credited to the grains group and the sugar would be credited (in teaspoon equivalents) to added sugars under discretionary calories. With this system, some food mixtures make small contributions to one or more food groups and make proportionately larger contributions to discretionary calories. Peach pie, for example, provides fruit that is credited to the fruit group and flour that is credited to the grains group, but the sugar and shortening would be credited to discretionary calories.

To obtain the disaggregated food-level data needed to estimate MyPyramid food group intakes, the authors of the 2008 Diet Quality Report linked the foods reported in NHANES 24-hour recalls to the *MyPyramid Equivalents Database for USDA Survey Food Codes* (USDA, 2006b). That database contains values for the MyPyramid food groups and subgroups (as described above) for every food reported in NHANES 1999–2002, as well as values for oils, solid fats, and added sugars.[7] The values for fruit, vegetables, milk, and milk products are reported in cup equivalents; and those for grains and for meats and beans are reported in ounce

[5]Note the emphasis on foods with no added sugars or fats, lean meats, and fat-free milk.
[6]Hereafter, the meat and meat alternateves group is called the meat and beans group for convenience.
[7]Alcohol is also counted under discretionary calories but is omitted from this report on the Nutrition Standards for school meals.

equivalents. Discretionary calories are reported in grams of solid fats and teaspoons of added sugars.

The committee compared the published values for children's mean intakes of MyPyramid food groups to MyPyramid food intake patterns for specific calorie levels. The calorie levels chosen (1,600 calories for children ages 6–8 years, 2,000 calories for children ages 9–13 years, and 2,400 calories from children ages 14–18 years) were based on the Estimated Energy Requirements (EERs) reported in SNDA-III. These requirements are discussed under *Energy* later in this chapter.

Results and Discussion

Figure 4-1 illustrates graphically how children's one day intakes compared with the MyPyramid food guidance system recommendations. For all age groups, the level of consumption of total grains was high and the level of consumption of whole grains and the three types of vegetables combined was very low.

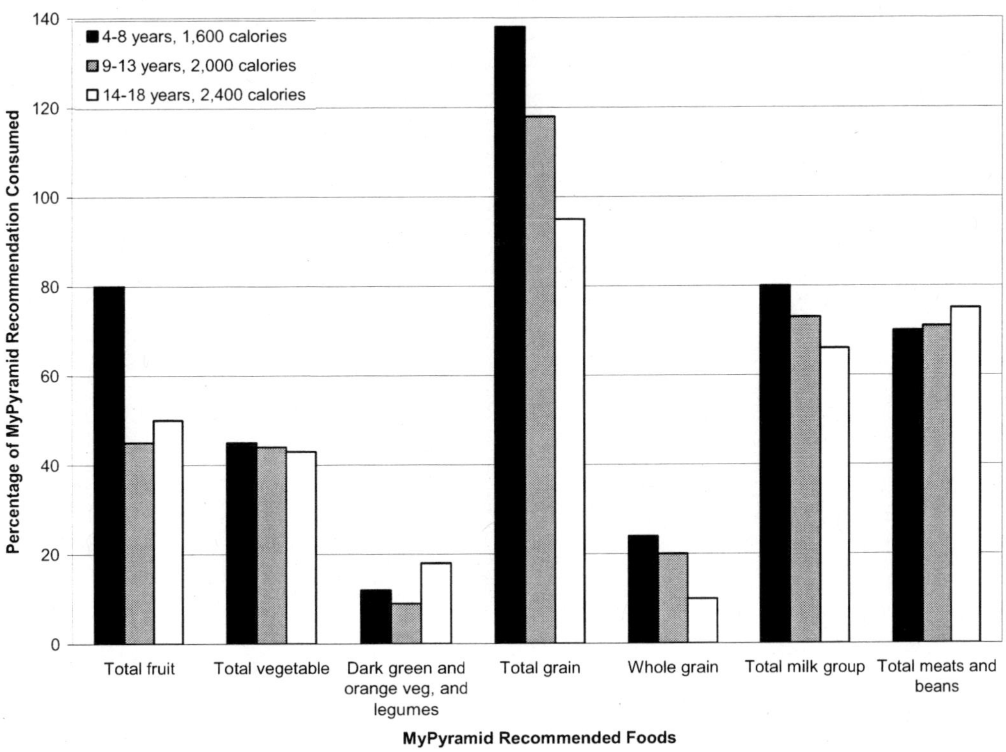

FIGURE 4-1 Percentages of MyPyramid recommended food groups or food components consumed, by age group, based on the recommended daily amounts for the specified level of calories.
NOTE: veg = vegetable.
SOURCE: USDA, 2008l.

Tables 4-2 through 4-4 compare the reported mean daily amounts of each MyPyramid food group consumed with the MyPyramid pattern for the specified calorie level. Data are presented in the three tables for the following age groups, respectively: 5–8 years, 9–13 years, and 14–18 years. Data are not presented by gender because these data were not available in the 2008 Diet Quality Report. Also in that report, the data for three vegetable subgroups (dark green vegetables, orange vegetables, and legumes) were combined; therefore, the analysis reflects these vegetables as one group.

For children ages 5–8 years, the mean level of grain consumption reported was 38 percent higher than the MyPyramid recommendation. However, few of the grains that children consumed were whole grains. The mean level of consumption of whole grains was less than one-fourth of the MyPyramid recommendation. The mean intakes reported were about 80 percent of the amounts recommended for the fruit and milk groups and 70 percent of the amounts recommended for the meats and beans group. The mean level of intake of vegetables was low—less than half the recommended amount—and the levels of consumption of dark green and orange vegetables and legumes were especially low.

TABLE 4-2 Mean Daily Amounts of MyPyramid Food Groups Consumed Compared with a 1,600-Calorie MyPyramid Food Intake Pattern, Children Ages 5–8 Years

Food Group or Component	MyPyramid Food Intake Pattern of 1,600 Calories	Mean Daily Consumption	Percentage of the MyPyramid Food Recommendation Consumed
Total fruit (cup equiv)	1.5	1.2	80
Total vegetables (cup equiv)	2	0.9	45
Dark green and orange vegetables and legumes	0.86[a]	0.1	12
Total grains (oz equiv)	5	6.9	138
Whole grains (oz equiv)	2.5[b]	0.6	24
Total milk group (oz equiv)	3	2.4	80
Total meats and beans (oz equiv)	5	3.5	70

NOTE: The sample (n = 578) included schoolchildren, and weekday food consumption recalls were obtained during periods when school was in session. Estimates are based on a single 24-hour recall per child. The MyPyramid food intake pattern used is from the *Dietary Guidelines for Americans* (HHS/USDA, 2005). equiv = equivalent; oz = ounces.

[a]Based on the recommendation of 6 cup equivalents per week.

[b]Based on the recommendation that half of all grain equivalents be whole grains.

SOURCE: Weighted tabulations of data from NHANES 1999–2002, as reported in *Diet Quality of American School-Age Children by School Lunch Participation Status* (USDA, 2008l); adapted from Table C-20.

The mean intakes of vegetables, grains, and meats and beans reported by children ages 9–13 years were comparable to those reported by younger children (Table 4-3). However, the mean intake of fruits was considerably lower, and the mean intake of milk and milk products was somewhat lower. Children ages 9–13 years consumed less than half (45 percent) the recommended amount of fruit and 71 percent of the recommended amount of milk and milk products.

TABLE 4-3 Mean Daily Amounts of MyPyramid Food Groups Consumed Compared with a 2,000-Calorie MyPyramid Food Intake Pattern, Children Ages 9–13 Years

Food Group or Component	MyPyramid Food Intake Pattern of 2,000 calories	Mean Daily Consumption	Percentage of the MyPyramid Food Recommendation Consumed
Total fruit (cup equiv)	2	0.9	45
Total vegetables (cup equiv)	2.5	1.1	44
Dark green and orange vegetables and legumes	1.14[a]	0.1	9
Total grains (oz equiv)	6	7.1	118
Whole grains (oz equiv)	3[b]	0.6	20
Total milk group (oz equiv)	3	2.2	73
Total meat and bean (oz equiv)	5.5	3.9	71

NOTE: The sample ($n = 998$) included schoolchildren, and weekday food consumption recalls were provided during periods when school was in session. Excludes pregnant and breast-feeding females. Estimates are based on a single 24-hour recall per child. The MyPyramid food intake pattern used is from the *Dietary Guidelines for Americans* (HHS/USDA, 2005). equiv = equivalent; oz = ounce.

[a]Based on the recommendation of 6 cup equivalents per week.

[b]Based on the recommendation that half of all grain equivalents be whole grains.

SOURCE: Weighted tabulations of data from NHANES 1999–2002, as reported in *Diet Quality of American School-Age Children by School Lunch Participation Status* (USDA, 2008l); adapted from Table C-20.

Finally, the findings for children ages 14–18 years were similar to those reported for younger children, but the mean intakes generally represented somewhat smaller percentages of the recommended amounts (Table 4-4). The only food group for which the mean intake exceeded 80 percent of the recommendation was grains.

TABLE 4-4 Mean Daily Amounts of MyPyramid Food Groups Consumed Compared with 2,400-Calorie MyPyramid Food Intake Pattern, Children Ages 14–18 Years

Food Group or Component	MyPyramid Food Intake Pattern of 2,400 calories	Mean Daily Consumption	Percentage of the MyPyramid Food Recommendation Consumed
Total fruit (cup equiv)	2	1	50
Total vegetables (cup equiv)	3	1.3	43
Dark green and orange vegetables and legumes	1.14[a]	0.2	18
Total grains (oz equiv)	8	7.6	95
Whole grains (oz equiv)	4[b]	0.4	10
Total milk group (oz equiv)	3	2	66
Total meats and bean (oz equiv)	6.5	4.9	75

NOTE: The sample (n = 1,021) included schoolchildren, and weekday food consumption recalls were obtained during periods when school was in session. Excludes pregnant and breast-feeding females. Estimates are based on a single 24-hour recall per child. The MyPyramid food intake pattern used is from the *Dietary Guidelines for Americans* (HHS/USDA, 2005). equiv = equivalent; oz = ounce.

[a]Based on the recommendation of 6 cup equivalents per week.

[b]Based on the recommendation that half of all grain equivalents be whole grains.

SOURCE: Weighted tabulations of data from NHANES 1999–2002, as reported in *Diet Quality of American School-Age Children by School Lunch Participation Status* (USDA, 2008l); adapted from Table C-20.

The *Dietary Guidelines for Americans* recommend that the majority of fruit intake come from whole fruits (fresh, frozen, canned, or dried) rather than fruit juice. Data presented in the 2008 Diet Quality Report indicate that whole fruits accounted for about 40 to 50 percent of children's total fruit intakes (USDA, 2008l).

Children consumed excessive amounts of discretionary calories from solid fats and added sugars,[8] as shown in Table 4-5. On average, the food intakes reported by schoolchildren included 2.6 to 5.5 times the recommended number of discretionary calories from these sources. The top five contributors to discretionary solid fat in the diets of schoolchildren were sandwiches (other than burgers), french fries and other fried potato products, pizza with meat, whole milk, and hamburgers and cheeseburgers (USDA, 2008l). The leading contributors to added discretionary sugars were regular sodas, noncarbonated sweetened drinks, candy, ready-to-eat breakfast cereals, and ice cream.

TABLE 4-5 Mean Daily Intakes of Discretionary Calories from Solid Fats and Added Sugars, by Age Group

Parameter	5–8 years (n = 578)	9–13 years (n = 998)	14–18 years (n = 1,021)
Calorie level for age group	1,600	2,000	2,400
MyPyramid discretionary calorie allowance	132	267	362
Mean intake of discretionary solid fat			
Grams	44.4	47.4	51.2
Calories[a]	400	427	461
Mean intake of discretionary added sugars			
Teaspoons	19	22.8	28.9
Calories[b]	319	383	486
Total discretionary calories			
Mean	719	810	947
Mean percent of discretionary calorie allowance	545	303	262

NOTE: n = sample size.

[a]Estimated on the basis of the number of grams (g) of discretionary solid fat (fat g × 9 calories/g).

[b]Estimated on the basis of the number of teaspoons (tsp) of added sugars (tsp × 4.2 g/tsp × 4 calories/g).

SOURCES: Weighted tabulations of data from NHANES 1999–2002, as reported in *Diet Quality of American School-Age Children by School Lunch Participation Status* (USDA, 2008l); adapted from Table C-20. Sample includes schoolchildren with weekday recalls during periods when school was in session. Excludes pregnant and breastfeeding females. Estimates are based on a single 24-hour recall per child. MyPyramid discretionary calorie allowance used was from *Dietary Guidelines for Americans* (HHS/USDA, 2005).

[8]Discretionary calorie intake is also influenced by the consumption of more than the recommended amounts of MyPyramid food groups, as was observed for grain intakes of children ages 5–8 years and 9–13 years (Tables 4-2 and 4-3).

Summary of Food Intakes

The findings presented above show that all children from age 5 through 18 years had mean intakes of vegetables, fruits, meats, whole grains, and milk that were less than the MyPyramid recommendations. Notably, children's intake of discretionary calories from solid fat and added sugars was substantially higher than the amount specified in MyPyramid food intake patterns. In general, vegetable intakes were 50 percent or less than the specified amounts for all ages, and fruit intakes were 50 percent or less than the specified amounts for children ages 9–18 years. Moreover, for children ages 5–13 years, mean intake of total grains (mainly refined grains) exceeded recommended levels. Although these findings do not necessarily indicate that the children had inadequate intakes of some of the nutrient that these food groups provide, they indicate the kinds of dietary improvements that would improve consistency with the *Dietary Guidelines for Americans*.

ASSESSMENT OF NUTRIENT INTAKES

A primary focus of the committee's assessment of nutrients was to examine the apparent prevalence of inadequate or excessive intakes of nutrients. In its assessment, the committee examined data that compared the distributions of usual nutrient intakes to the DRIs developed by the Institute of Medicine of The National Academies (IOM, 1997, 1998, 2000a, 2001, 2002/2005, 2005). These data were obtained from the 2008 Diet Quality Report (USDA, 2008l) and the SNDA-III report (USDA, 2007a). Both of these reports used methods recommended by the Institute of Medicine (IOM, 2000b) to estimate usual intake distributions and to apply the DRIs.

Estimating Usual Nutrient Intakes

The usual intake of a nutrient is an individual's long-term average intake of that nutrient (NRC, 1986). Usual intake must be estimated; it cannot be observed, because day-to-day intakes vary considerably. The Iowa State University Method (Nusser et al., 1996) is the commonly used and accepted approach for estimating the usual intakes by population groups. This method estimates the distribution of usual intakes by using a single 24-hour recall for all members of the group and a second 24-hour recall for some proportion of the group. In SNDA-III, the personal computer version of the Software for Intake Distribution Estimation (PC-SIDE; ISU, 1997) was used to estimate (1) usual nutrient intake distributions and (2) the proportion of children with usual intakes above or below the defined cutoff values. Based on procedures recommended by the Institute of Medicine (IOM, 2000), a random subsample of children (666 of the 2,314 children who completed the Day 1 recall) provided the required second 24-hour recalls. Comparable methods were used in the 2008 Diet Quality Report to analyze data from NHANES 1999–2004 (see Appendix I).

Applying the Dietary Reference Intakes: Institute of Medicine Methodology

The DRIs released by the Institute of Medicine replaced the previously used RDAs (NRC, 1989) as authoritative reference values. The DRIs provide six different types of reference values for use in the assessment and planning of diets. These include the Estimated Average Requirement (EAR), AI for nutrients without an EAR, the RDA, the UL, the Acceptable

Macronutrient Distribution Range (AMDR), and the EER. Contrary to earlier practice, all except the RDAs are useful for the assessment of nutrient intakes. The RDAs are inappropriate for the assessment of the nutrient intakes of groups, because the percentage of individuals below the RDA is not a true estimate of the percentage of individuals with inadequate intakes. Only a method that considers the full distribution of requirements can estimate the prevalence of inadequacy. The EAR cut-point method, a short-cut of the full probability approach, may be used to obtain such an estimate (IOM, 2006). Consequently, estimation of the prevalence of nutrient inadequacy in a group by determining the proportion of individuals with intakes below the RDAs leads to an overestimation of the true prevalence of nutrient inadequacy (IOM, 2006b).

DRIs are defined for 12 different life-stage and gender groups. For schoolchildren, the groups are 5–8 years (both genders), males ages 9–13 years, females ages 9–13 years, males ages 14–18 years, and females ages 14–18 years.

Estimated Average Requirement

An EAR is the usual daily intake level that is estimated to meet the nutrient requirements of half of the healthy individuals in a life-stage and gender group. The proportion of a group with usual daily intakes below the EAR is an estimate of the prevalence of nutrient inadequacy in that population group. With the exception of iron for female adolescents, the method of choice for assessment of the prevalence of nutrient inadequacy is the EAR cut-point method (IOM, 2001, 2003). The EAR cut-point method involves estimation of the proportion of individuals in a group whose usual nutrient intakes are less than the EAR. It has been shown that under certain assumptions, the proportion with usual intakes less than the EAR is an estimate of the proportion of a group whose usual intakes do not meet the requirements (Beaton, 1994; Carriquiry, 1999; IOM, 2000b). This approach was used in the studies for both the 2008 Diet Quality Report and the SNDA-III report to estimate the prevalence of inadequate intakes of protein, carbohydrates, nine vitamins (A, B_6, B_{12}, C, E, thiamin, riboflavin, niacin, and folate), and three minerals (phosphorus, magnesium, and zinc) among schoolchildren.

For female adolescents, the probability approach (NRC, 1986) was used to assess iron intake, as recommended by the Institute of Medicine (IOM, 2001). This more complex approach accounts for both the distribution of iron requirements (which is skewed for this age-gender group; see IOM, 2001) and the distribution of usual intakes. *Dietary Reference Intakes: Applications in Dietary Assessment* (IOM, 2000b) provides more detailed information about these two methods.

Adequate Intake

When the evidence was insufficient to determine an EAR for a nutrient, the Institute of Medicine set AI values instead. The AI is defined as a recommended average daily nutrient intake level and is based on observed or experimentally derived intake levels or approximations of the mean nutrient intake level by a group (or groups) of apparently healthy people that are assumed to be adequate (IOM, 2006). As described by the Institute of Medicine (IOM, 2000b), the inherent limitations of the AI affect the inferences that can be made about the prevalence of inadequacy for nutrients with an AI (IOM, 2000b). The 2008 Diet Quality Report and SNDA-III provided data on children's intakes of calcium, potassium, fiber, linoleic acid, and linolenic acid by comparing the estimated mean intakes with the AI. Groups with mean intakes at or above the AI can generally be assumed to have a low prevalence of inadequacy for the criterion of adequate nutritional status used for that nutrient. Assumptions about the inadequacy of intakes cannot be made when the mean intake is below the AI.

Tolerable Upper Intake Levels

A UL is the highest daily intake level that likely poses no risk of adverse health effects. As the usual daily intake increases above the UL, the risk of adverse effects increases. The ULs for most nutrients are based on intakes from supplements as well as intakes from foods and beverages. Neither the data from NHANES 1999–2004 that was analyzed for the 2008 Diet Quality Report nor the SNDA-III data include contributions from dietary supplements. For this reason, the committee's assessment of usual nutrient intakes relative to ULs focused on the intake of sodium.

Acceptable Macronutrient Distribution Range

AMDRs are defined for energy-providing macronutrients. AMDRs define a range of usual daily intakes that is associated with a reduced risk of chronic disease while providing AIs of essential nutrients. AMDRs are expressed as a percentage of the total energy intake. For example, the AMDR for fat for children ages 4 through 18 years is 25 to 35 percent of the total energy intake. The 2008 Diet Quality Report and SNDA-III provide data on the proportions of children with usual intakes of protein, carbohydrates, total fat, linoleic acid, and linolenic acid that fell within defined AMDRs, as well as proportions with usual intakes that exceeded and that fell below the AMDRs.

Estimated Energy Requirement

The EER is used to assess energy intakes. For children, the EER represents the sum of the dietary energy intake predicted to maintain energy balance for the child's age, weight, height, and activity level, plus an amount to cover normal growth and development. There is a distribution of EERs for groups of children, just as there is a distribution of usual intakes. The two distributions should have approximately equal mean values. SNDA-III provides data on the distributions of EERs and on the distributions of usual energy intakes. The 2008 Diet Quality Report does not estimate EERs.

Saturated Fat and Cholesterol

DRIs are not defined for saturated fat and cholesterol. The dietary guidance given in the DRIs recommends that the levels of consumption of saturated fat and cholesterol be as low as possible while consuming a nutritionally adequate diet (IOM, 2002/2005). Because the 2005 *Dietary Guidelines for Americans* provide recommendations concerning saturated fat and cholesterol, the committee included these food components in its assessment children's usual nutrient intakes. Both the 2008 Diet Quality Report and SNDA-III provide data on the proportions of children whose usual intakes of saturated fat and cholesterol exceeded the maximum intakes recommended.

Results and Discussion

In considering estimates of children's usual nutrient intakes, emphasis is given to the data from SNDA-III. This emphasis is motivated by four factors. First, the SNDA-III data were collected more recently than the NHANES data that were included in the 2008 Diet Quality

Report (the 2004–2005 school year and the years 1999 through 2004, respectively). Second, all of the 24-hour recalls included in SNDA-III reflect days when the children were in school. The 2008 Diet Quality Report attempted to restrict the sample in this way (see Appendix I), but 24-hour recalls for some children may cover days when they did not attend school. Third, as described previously, SNDA-III includes specific data collection strategies to minimize reporting errors among young children. Fourth, SNDA-III collected detailed information about the foods and beverages offered in school meals and used these data to generate estimates of the nutrient contents of foods that children consumed as part of school meals. As such, the SNDA-III data provide the best estimates of the usual nutrient intakes by U.S. schoolchildren on school days.

An important note is that the NHANES data from the 2008 Diet Quality Report lead to qualitatively similar conclusions about the adequacy and the potential excesses of children's usual nutrient intakes (specific point estimates may vary). The same is true for the NHANES data from 1999 through 2004 on the usual intakes by U.S. children that are not restricted to school days. These data were reported in a separate volume of the 2008 Diet Quality Report that focused on Food Stamp program participants and nonparticipants (USDA, 2008o). Key tabulations from both of these data sets are provided on the Food and Nutrition Service website (http://www.fns.usda.gov/oane).

Tables 4-6 through 4-10 summarize the SNDA-III data on the usual nutrient intakes by schoolchildren relative to the DRIs and the 2005 *Dietary Guidelines for Americans*. Individual point estimates in these tables may be statistically unreliable because of a small sample size or a large coefficient of variation. In reporting percentages at the extreme, the committee used the convention developed by Moshfegh et al. (USDA/ARS, 2005) in reporting usual nutrient intake data for the population, as noted in the tables.

Data on mean intakes and the full distributions of usual intakes (5th, 10th, 25th, 50th, 75th, 90th, and 95th percentiles) are available for National School Lunch Program participants and nonparticipants and for all children at http://www.fns.usda.gov/oane. That site presents data for each of the age and gender subgroups covered in Tables 4-6 through 4-10, which follow.

Nutrients with Estimated Average Requirements

Results For the youngest schoolchildren (6–8 years), the estimated prevalence of inadequacy was very low (<3 percent) for all nutrients examined other than vitamin E (Table 4-6). For older children, particularly females, the prevalence of inadequacy exceeded 10 percent for several nutrients. Key findings are summarized below, followed by a brief discussion.

- **Magnesium** More than 70 percent of adolescents (14–18 years) had inadequate usual intakes of magnesium. The prevalence of inadequacy was lower among children ages 9–13 years but ranged from about 12 percent for males to 29 percent for females.
- **Vitamin A** Almost half (49 percent) of males ages 14–18 years and 58 percent of females ages 14–18 years had inadequate usual intakes of vitamin A. Among children ages 9–13 years, the prevalence of inadequacy ranged from about 13 to 22 percent and was the highest among females.
- **Phosphorus** Almost half (46 percent) of females ages 14–18 years and more than a quarter (28 percent) of females ages 9–13 years had inadequate usual intakes of phosphorus. The prevalence of inadequacy was substantially lower (less than 10 percent) for males in these age groups.
- **Zinc** A similar pattern of differences by gender was observed for the adequacy of the zinc intake. More than a quarter (28 percent) of females ages 14–18 years and about 12 percent

of females ages 9–13 years had inadequate intakes of zinc, whereas less than 10 percent of males had inadequate intakes of zinc.

- **Vitamin C** Among adolescents ages 14–18 years, 40 percent of females and 27 percent of males had inadequate usual intakes of vitamin C. The prevalence of inadequacy was lower among children ages 9–13 years, especially males; 13 percent of females in this age group had inadequate intakes of vitamin C.
- **Other vitamins and nutrients** For several other vitamins and nutrients, the prevalence of inadequate intakes was high for adolescent females (14–18 years), but rare for other age-gender subgroups.

TABLE 4-6 Estimated Prevalence of Inadequacy of Selected Vitamins, Minerals, Protein, and Carbohydrate Among Schoolchildren Based on Usual Nutrient Intakes from SNDA-III[a]

	Estimated Prevalence of Inadequate Usual Intakes (%)				
Nutrient	6–8 yr, both genders (n = 343)	9–13 yr, males (n = 469)	9–13 yr, females (n = 484)	14–18 yr, males (n = 506)	14–18 yr, females (n = 512)
Vitamin A	<3[b]	13*	22	49	58
Vitamin C	<3	4*	13*	27	40
Vitamin E	64	87	91	95	>97[c]
Vitamin B_6	<3	<3	<3	<3	20
Vitamin B_{12}	<3	<3	<3	<3	12*
Folate	<3	<3	<3	<3	24
Niacin	<3	<3	<3	<3	9*
Riboflavin	<3	<3	<3	<3	7*
Thiamin	<3	<3	<3	3*	17
Iron	<3	<3	<3	<3	16
Magnesium	<3	12*	29	72	87
Phosphorus	<3	6*	28	9*	46
Zinc	<3	<3	12*	7*	28
Protein	<3	<3	3	<3	16
Carbohydrate	<3	<3	<3	<3	<3

NOTE: n = sample size; * = point estimate may not be reliable because of an inadequate cell size or a large coefficient of variation. <3 is reported in rare occurrences.

[a]Nutrients in this table have EARs.

[b]Less than 3 percent is reported in rare occurrences (less than 3 percent of students had usual intakes in this range, but the specific point estimates was statistically unreliable).

[c]More than 97 percent is report for common occurrences (more than 97 percent of students had usual intakes in this range, but the specific point estimate was statistically unreliable).

SOURCES: Weighted tabulations of data from SNDA-III (USDA, 2007a); adapted from Table VI.16 in Volume II and Table J.16 in Appendix J to Volume II. Dietary intake data (24-hour recalls) were collected during the 2004–2005 school year and do not include intakes from dietary supplements (e.g., multivitamin-multimineral preparations). The personal computer version of the Software for Intake Distribution Estimation (PC-SIDE; ISU, 1997) was used to estimate the usual nutrient intake distributions and the percentage of children with usual intakes below the EARs. The EARs used in the analysis were from the DRI reports (IOM, 1997, 1998, 2000a, 2001, 2002/2005).

Discussion Although available biochemical data indicate no measurable manifestations of deficiencies associated with magnesium, vitamin A, phosphorus, zinc, or vitamin C (CDC, 2008c), the outcomes of the analyses of the nutrient intake data are suggestive of food patterns that could be improved. However, at least some members of the school-age population have laboratory evidence of iron deficiency.[9] The most recent NHANES data (CDC, 2002) revealed that the prevalence of iron deficiency among children of both genders ages 6–11 years was 4 percent; and for males ages 12–15, it was 5 percent. For females ages 12–15 years, however, the prevalence was 9 percent.

In addition, an apparent 24 percent prevalence of inadequate intakes of folate for adolescent females may represent a risk for some of these young women. The Centers for Disease Control and Prevention estimates that 50 to 70 percent of neural tube defects, including spina bifida and anencephaly, can be prevented if a female consumes folic acid before conception and throughout the first trimester of her pregnancy (CDC, 2004).

The prevalence of vitamin E inadequacy was high for all groups of children (range was 64 percent to more than 97 percent). This finding is consistent with most recent studies of vitamin E intake (USDA/ERS, 2007b). Devaney et al. (2004) noted that vitamin E intakes were inadequate even when dietary supplements were included in the analysis. Furthermore, the committee recognizes, however, that the Dietary Guidelines Advisory Committee accepted the DRIs for vitamin E (HHS/USDA, 2004) and, in turn, *Dietary Guidelines for Americans* states that vitamin E may be a nutrient of concern because of low intakes (HHS/USDA, 2005). The committee is aware, however, that the current vitamin E requirements are considered high by some and that clinical vitamin E deficiency is rare. The committee will continue to consider this issue during Phase II.

[9]Iron deficiency is defined as an abnormal value for at least two of the following three indicators: serum ferritin, transferrin saturation, and free erythrocyte protoporphyrin (CDC, 2002).

Nutrients with Adequate Intakes

For calcium, potassium, fiber, and vitamin D, the DRIs specify AIs rather than EARs. Table 4-7 presents data on the schoolchildren's mean intakes of all of these nutrients except vitamin D, which is discussed later in this section. As emphasized by the Institute of Medicine (IOM, 2000b), inherent limitations in the AI reference value affect conclusions that can be drawn about nutrient adequacy. If the usual mean intake is equal to or higher than the AI, the prevalence of inadequacy is likely to be low. If the usual mean intake is less than the AI, no firm conclusions can be drawn about the adequacy of usual intakes. However, when mean intakes are substantially lower than the AIs, there may be reason to be concerned about inadequacy.

TABLE 4-7 AIs and Mean Reported Usual Intakes of Calcium, Potassium, and Fiber of Schoolchildren on the Basis of Usual Nutrient Intakes from SNDA-III

Nutrient	6–8 yr, both genders (*n* = 343)	9–13 yr, males (*n* = 469)	9–13 yr, females (*n* = 484)	14–18 yr, males (*n* = 506)	14–18 yr, females (*n* = 512)
Calcium (mg)					
AI	800	1,300	1,300	1,300	1,300
Mean usual intake	1,093	1,213	1,050	1,248	847
Potassium (mg)					
AI	3,800	4,500	4,500	4,700	4,700
Mean usual intake	2,415	2,662	2,370	3,004	2,084
Fiber (g)					
AI	25	31	26	38	26
Mean usual intake	13.9	15	13.3	16.2	12
Fiber (g/1,000 kcal)					
AI	14	14	14	14	14
Mean usual intake	7.1	6.8	6.9	6.2	6.9

NOTE: g = grams; kcal = calories; mg = milligrams; *n* = sample size.

SOURCES: Weighted tabulations of data from the SNDA-III (USDA, 2007a); adapted from Table VI.16 in Volume II. Dietary intake data (24-hour recalls) were collected during the 2004–2005 school year and do not include intakes from dietary supplements (e.g., multivitamin-multimineral preparations). The personal computer version of the Software for Intake Distribution Estimation (PC-SIDE; ISU, 1997) was used to estimate usual nutrient intake distributions. The AIs used in the analysis were from the DRI reports (IOM, 1997, 2002/2005, 2005).

Calcium For calcium, the mean usual intake by children ages 6–8 years was higher than the AI, indicating that the prevalence of inadequate calcium intakes in this age group is likely to be low. The mean usual intakes of calcium for all groups of older children were lower than their respective AIs. The gap between the mean usual intake and the AI of calcium was larger for females than for males.

Inadequate calcium intake can constitute a notable health concern for schoolchildren. Peak bone mass is largely accrued during adolescence, and may not be achieved if optimal calcium intake is not reached. On average, the age of peak calcium accrual for females is reached at 12.5 years, while the age of peak accrual for males is 14 years old. Several studies support a potential relationship between low calcium intakes and fractures during adolescence (Goulding et al., 1998, 2001; Wyshak and Frisch, 1994). The risks of not attaining peak bone mass during adolescence include osteoporosis and bone fractures later in life (Greer et al., 2006; IOM, 1997).

Potassium For potassium, the mean usual intakes by all groups of children were lower than their respective AIs. Direct evidence on the potassium requirements of children is lacking (IOM, 2005). Because the conditions resulting from inadequate potassium intake are chronic and likely to result from inadequate intake over an extended period of time, there may be good reasons for concern about the current levels of potassium intake by children even in the face of limited data.

Fiber The level used to establish AIs for fiber was 14 grams per 1,000 calories (IOM, 2002/2005), which is based on the median energy intake of specific age-gender subgroups, as estimated from the 1994–1996, 1998 Continuing Survey of Food Intakes by Individuals. On a gram-per-1,000 calorie basis, children's usual daily fiber intakes were generally less than half of the 14 grams assumed in setting the AI. For all groups, even the 95th percentile of the distribution of usual fiber intake was less than the AI (see http://www.fns.usda.gov/oane). Part of the discrepancy is due to the fact that AIs are defined for total fiber (dietary fiber plus functional fiber), but food composition databases include values only for dietary fiber and do not include all sources of functional fiber. Thus, fiber intakes are underestimated, but not to an extent that would alleviate the marked disparities between the AIs and the usual intakes apparent in these data.[10] For this reason, some have suggested that the methods used to establish the AIs for fiber may need to be reexamined, especially for children and adolescents (USDA/ERS, 2007b).[11] The Institute of Medicine (IOM, 2002/2005) has concluded that the consumption of fiber should be increased to promote normal laxation, help prevent diet-related cancer, help reduce serum cholesterol concentrations and therefore the risk of coronary heart disease, and help prevent obesity and the risk of adult-onset diabetes.

Vitamin D Data on the vitamin D intake of schoolchildren are not available. Neither of the published analyses of usual nutrient intakes reviewed by the committee includes data on vitamin D intakes. Release 20 of USDA's National Nutrient Database for Standard Reference, the authoritative source of food composition data in the United States, contains vitamin D contents of only about 600 foods, whereas the vitamin C content of about 1,100 foods is listed (USDA/ARS, 2008). That database does not yet include the vitamin D contents of foods that have recently been fortified with vitamin D or the contents of specific forms of vitamin D. The challenges associated with the estimation of vitamin D intakes have been described by Yetley

[10]It is estimated that adults consume about 5.1 more grams per day of fiber than the amount estimated from current food composition databases (IOM, 2002/2005).

[11]The data used to establish AIs are drawn from studies of coronary heart disease risk among adults. Moreover, the AIs for children are two to three times higher than the standard previously used to assess fiber intake in this age group (USDA/ERS, 2007b).

(2008). Yetley (2008) has reviewed the results of selected vitamin D status assessments that were based on NHANES data. Those data have included serum 25-hydroxyvitamin D concentrations since 1988. Using existing reference values, the prevalence of low 25-hydroxyvitamin D (≤25.5 nanomoles per liter) for children was ≤1 percent for children ages 5–11 years and 5 percent for children ages 12–19 years. Nonetheless, the committee is aware of recent interest in reviewing and, if needed, updating the reference values associated with vitamin D as well as reviewing discussions about the appropriateness of 25-hydroxyvitamin D as a biomarker for vitamin D status. In September 2008, the Institute of Medicine put in place a new DRI study to review emerging data about vitamin D requirements and health. The relevance of newer information on vitamin D to the school meal programs must await the outcome of this important work.

Energy

The adequacy of usual energy intake may be evaluated by comparing energy intake estimates derived from self-reported food intake with EERs. Adipose tissue stores may also be used to evaluate the adequacy of usual energy intake, with excessive stores a marker for excessive energy intake and low stores indicative of chronic insufficient energy intake. This can be assessed by examining the prevalence of obesity and underweight, as discussed in Chapters 1 and 2, respectively.

The assessment of self-reported energy intakes is challenging. In theory, populations that are in energy balance (not gaining or losing weight) should have average usual energy intakes that are roughly equivalent to their corresponding EERs. However, as noted earlier, it is well recognized that children or their caregivers tend to misreport food intake in dietary surveys. The accurate estimation of EERs also requires accurate information about customary levels of physical activity. Rather than collecting detailed data about physical activity, SNDA-III assumes a "low active" level of physical activity for all children. The study's authors used this assumption because data from the Youth Media Campaign Longitudinal Survey indicate that relatively few children are engaged in regular physical activity (USDA, 2007a). The survey found that more than 60 percent of children ages 9 through 13 years did not participate in any organized physical activity during their non-school hours and that about 23 percent did not engage in physical activity during their free time (CDC, 2003).

Reported usual energy intakes and EERs for schoolchildren are shown in Table 4-8.[12] For children ages 6–8 years and females ages 9–13 years, both the mean and median reported usual energy intakes exceeded the mean and median EERs. The gap was approximately 400 calories for the youngest children and approximately 200 calories for the older females. Excess daily usual energy intakes in this range would lead to an annual weight gain of approximately 20 to 30 pounds. The magnitude of the difference between usual energy intake and the EER suggests that the food intakes for these age groups were overreported. However, an alternative explanation for the discrepancy between mean usual energy intakes and mean EERs is that EERs were underestimated because a low-active level of physical activity was assumed for all children (USDA, 2007a).

In contrast, for adolescents ages 14–18 years, reported usual energy intakes were less than the EERs. For males, the mean reported energy intake was roughly 300 calories less than the

[12]Compared with the findings from SNDA-III, the mean usual energy intakes reported in the 2008 Diet Quality Report, based on data from the NHANES 1999–2004 (USDA, 2008l), were comparable for the youngest children (mean of 1,912 calories for children ages 5–8 years) and somewhat lower for females ages 9–13 years (1,898 calories) (see http://www.fns.usda.gov/oane).

corresponding EER. The discrepancy was smaller for females (130 calories).[13] These findings may reflect a tendency for adolescents to underreport food intakes.

TABLE 4-8 Reported Usual Food Energy Intakes and EERs

Parameter	6–8 yr, both genders (*n* = 343)	9–13 yr, males (*n* = 469)	9–13 yr, females (*n* = 484)	9–13 yr, both genders	14–18 yr, males (*n* = 506)	14–18 yr, females (*n* = 512)	14–18 yr, both genders
Usual energy intake (kcal/day)							
Median	1,944	2,203	1,923	2,060	2,570	1,772	2,129
Mean	1,968	2,239	1,960	2,103	2,625	1,830	2,214
EER (kcal/day)							
Median	1,527	2,117	1,724	1,873	2,782	1,923	2,261
Mean	1,574	2,223	1,752	1,993	2,874	1,960	2,411

NOTE: kcal = calories; *n* = sample size.
SOURCES: Weighted tabulations of data from the SNDA-III (USDA, 2007a); adapted from Tables J.1a and J.1b in Appendix J to Volume II of the report. Dietary intake data (24-hour recalls) were collected during the 2004–2005 school year. The personal computer version of the Software for Intake Distribution Estimation (PC-SIDE; ISU, 1997) was used to estimate usual nutrient intake distributions. EERs were calculated by using algorithms defined in *Dietary Reference Intakes: Applications in Dietary Assessment* (IOM, 2000b) and by assuming a low-active level of physical activity.

[13]Compared with the findings from SNDA-III, the mean usual energy intakes reported in the 2008 Diet Quality Report, based on data from NHANES 1999–2004 (USDA, 2008l), were comparable for males (mean equals 2,635 calories) and higher for females (mean equals 1,924 calories) ages 14–18 years (see http://www.fns.usda.gov/oane).

In any case, data in Chapter 1 make it clear that obesity is a growing concern for schoolchildren; and, therefore, excessive energy intake is a major concern. During Phase II, the committee will consider the levels of calories in the overall diet of schoolchildren and appropriate calorie levels for the Nutrition Standards and Meal Requirements for school meals.

Macronutrients

Information on macronutrient intake relative to the AMDRs is shown in Table 4-9. All schoolchildren had usual intakes of protein, as a percentage of total energy intake, that were consistent with the AMDR, which is 10 to 30 percent of total energy. With the exception of adolescent females, the same was true for usual intakes of carbohydrate. Five percent of adolescent females had usual carbohydrate intakes that exceeded the upper bound of the AMDR (which is 45 to 65 percent of total energy), and about 8 percent had usual carbohydrate intakes that fell below the lower bound of the AMDR.

TABLE 4-9 Percentage of Schoolchildren with Reported Usual Intakes of Macronutrients Outside the AMDR Range, Based on Usual Nutrient Intakes from SNDA-III

Nutrient	6–8 yr, both genders (*n* = 343)	9–13 yr, males (*n* = 469)	9–13 yr, females (*n* = 484)	14–18 yr, males (*n* = 506)	14–18 yr, females (*n* = 512)
Carbohydrate					
Greater than AMDR	<3[a]	<3	<3	<3	5
Less than AMDR	<3	<3	<3	<3	8.2
Protein					
Greater than AMDR	<3	<3	<3	<3	<3
Less than AMDR	<3	<3	<3	<3	<3
Total fat					
Greater than AMDR	18.6	<3	11	22.2	31.4
Less than AMDR	<3	<3	<3	<3	9.3

NOTE: *n* = sample size; * = point estimate may not be reliable because of an inadequate cell size or a large coefficient of variation.

[a]Less than 3 percent is reported in rare occurrences (less than 3 percent of students had usual intakes in this range, but the specific point estimates was statistically unreliable).

SOURCES: Weighted tabulations of data from SNDA-III (USDA, 2007a); adapted from Tables J.3, J.15, and J.17 in Appendix J to Volume II. Dietary intake data (24-hour recalls) were collected during the 2004–2005 school year. The personal computer version of the Software for Intake Distribution Estimation (PC-SIDE; ISU, 1997) was used to estimate usual nutrient intake distributions and the percentage of children with usual intakes outside the reference value(s). The AMDRs used in the analysis were from the macronutrient DRI report (IOM, 2002/2005).

More than 60 percent of children in all age groups had usual fat intakes that were within the AMDR (25 to 35 percent of total calories). As shown in Table 4-9, the intakes for the majority of children whose usual fat intakes were outside the AMDR exceeded the upper bound of the range.

During Phase II, the committee will consider both the total amount and the nature of the types of fats that are appropriate for the Nutrition Standards and Meal Requirements for the school meal programs.

Excessive Intakes

Nutrients with Tolerable Upper Levels of Intake Because supplement data were unavailable, it generally was not possible to determine whether nutrients were consumed in amounts that were higher than the UL. Sodium is the primary nutrient that the committee is considering with regard to the potential for exceeding the UL. The Institute of Medicine (IOM, 2005) has underscored the potential for excessive sodium intake to adversely affect blood pressure in children. However, overall, more than 90 percent of schoolchildren had usual sodium intake that exceeded the UL (see Table 4-10).

TABLE 4-10 Percentage of Schoolchildren with Reported Usual Intakes of Sodium that Exceeded the UL, Based on Usual Nutrient Intakes from SNDA-III

Parameter	6–8 yr, both genders (n = 343)	9–13 yr, males (n = 469)	9–13 yr, females (n = 484)	14–18 yr, males (n = 506)	14–18 yr, females (n = 512)
Sodium UL (g/day)	1.9	2.2	2.2	2.3	2.3
% Greater than UL	>97[a]	>97	90	>97	75

NOTE: g/day = grams per day; mg = milligrams; n = sample size.

[a]More than 97 percent is report for common occurrences (more than 97 percent of students had usual intakes in this range, but the specific point estimate was statistically unreliable).

SOURCES: Weighted tabulations of data from SNDA-III (USDA, 2007a); adapted from Table J.33 in Appendix J to Volume II. Dietary intake data (24-hour recalls) were collected during the 2004–2005 school year and do not include intake from dietary supplements. The personal computer version of the Software for Intake Distribution Estimation (PC-SIDE; ISU, 1997) was used to estimate usual nutrient intake distributions and the percentage of children with usual intakes that exceeded the reference value. The ULs used in the analysis were from two DRI reports (IOM, 2002/2005, 2005).

The committee compared the usual nutrient intake distributions of calcium, iron, phosphorus, and zinc (see http://www.fns.usda.gov/oane) with the defined ULs. The risk of excessive intakes from foods and beverages alone appears to be low for all these nutrients except zinc. For all the age-gender subgroups examined, intakes at the 95th percentile of the distribution were well below the ULs for all but one of these nutrients. For zinc, more than 25 percent of children ages 6–8 years had usual intakes that exceeded the UL (the UL is 12 grams and the intake at the 75th percentile of the distribution was 12.6 grams). For older children, zinc intakes at the 95th percentile of the distribution were below the UL.

Saturated fat and cholesterol Percentages of schoolchildren with reported usual intakes that exceed recommended limits for saturated fat and cholesterol, as specified by the 2005 *Dietary Guidelines for Americans*, are shown in Table 4-11.

TABLE 4-11 Percentages of Schoolchildren with Reported Usual Intakes that Exceed Recommended Limits for Saturated Fat and Cholesterol,[a] Based on Usual Nutrient Intakes from SNDA-III

Nutrient	6–8 yr, both genders (*n* =343)	9–13 yr, males (*n* =469)	9–13 yr, females (*n*=484)	14–18 yr, males (*n* =506)	14–18 yr, females (*n* =512)
Saturated Fat >10% of total food energy	78.7	89.5*	>97[b]	76.7	74.6
Cholesterol > 300 mg	4.8*	15.6*	<3[c]	36.6	9.0*

NOTE: * = point estimate may not be reliable because of an inadequate cell size or a large coefficient of variation.

[a]The reference values used for saturated fat and cholesterol are taken from *Dietary Guidelines for Americans* (HHS/USDA, 2005). The DRI guideline for saturated fat is to consume amounts as low as possible while consuming a nutritionally adequate diet (IOM, 2002/2005).

[b]More than 97 percent is report for common occurrences (more than 97 percent of students had usual intakes in this range, but the specific point estimate was statistically unreliable).

[c]Less than 3 percent is reported in rare occurrences (less than 3 percent of students had usual intakes in this range, but the specific point estimates was statistically unreliable).

SOURCES: Weighted tabulations of data from SNDA-III (USDA, 2007a); adapted from Tables J.5 and J.37 in Appendix J to Volume II. Dietary intake data (24-hour recalls) were collected during the 2004–2005 school year and do not include intake from dietary supplements. The personal computer version of the Software for Intake Distribution Estimation (PC-SIDE; ISU, 1997) was used to estimate usual nutrient intake distributions and the percentage of children with usual intakes that exceeded the reference value.

More than three-quarters of children in all age-gender subgroups had usual saturated fat intakes that exceeded the limit recommended in the 2005 *Dietary Guidelines for Americans* (HHS/USDA, 2005). More than 85 percent of all schoolchildren had usual cholesterol intakes that were consistent with the guidance. The prevalence of excessive cholesterol intakes was higher for males than for females and was highest among adolescent males. Appropriate amounts of these food substances will be considered during Phase II of this study.

***Trans* fatty acids** The DRIs do not include reference values for *trans* fatty acids, but the Institute of Medicine's recommendation is to keep intake as low as possible while consuming a nutritionally adequate diet (IOM, 2002/2005). The DRIs do not include reference values for *trans* fatty acids. *Dietary Guidelines for Americans* recommend limiting the intake of fats and oils containing *trans* fat. The committee could not estimate *trans* fat intake, however, because neither of the published studies reviewed by the committee includes data on this food component. *Trans* fatty acids are not included in the food and nutrient database used to analyze dietary recalls collected in NHANES and SNDA-III (USDA/ARS, 2004). Nonetheless, the requirement (as of January 1, 2006) that the *trans* fat content be listed on Nutrition Facts Labels would enable the committee to make feasible recommendations concerning the *trans* fat content of school meals.

Other

Substances found in food ranging from additives to contaminants to caffeine are often cited as factors to consider in planning meals for children. While not addressed specifically in this Phase I report, such substances may be considered during the Phase II deliberations, as appropriate and as feasible.

Summary of Nutrient Assessment

The findings presented in this chapter provide a picture of the prevalence of apparent nutrient inadequacies, the prevalence of the risk of excessive intakes, and dietary imbalances among schoolchildren. Although the data are based on estimates of intake and have important limitations, as described here, they provide a foundation for identifying those nutrients in the diets of schoolchildren that merit consideration during the Phase II deliberations. On the basis of the available intake data, concerns about inadequate intakes are the greatest for older children. However, the low prevalence of inadequacy estimated for younger children could be influenced by overreported food intakes. For adolescent females, the data suggest that the intakes of virtually all vitamins and minerals merit attention. However, the high prevalence of inadequate intakes estimated for adolescent females could be influenced by underreported food intakes.

The calcium intakes by children ages 6–8 years appear to be adequate. The mean and median calcium intakes by older children are less than the AI, and the gap is the highest for adolescents ages 14–18 years, especially females. The mean and median intakes of potassium and fiber were substantially lower than the AI for all groups of children. These findings suggest the potential for inadequate intakes of these nutrients. The total intakes of fiber are underestimated because of limitations in food composition data, and there may be problems with the existing AIs for fiber. However, the magnitude of the gap between the usual intakes and the AIs for fiber suggests that children's fiber intakes are inadequate.

The intakes of saturated fat are a major concern. More than three-quarters of children in all age and gender groups had usual saturated fat intakes that exceeded the recommendation of the

Dietary Guidelines for Americans of less than 10 percent of total energy. Total fat intake is of less concern. Nonetheless, the usual fat intakes by some children were excessive.

Finally, children's sodium intakes merit close attention. Three-quarters or more of children in all age groups had usual intakes of sodium that exceeded the UL, and in most cases, the prevalence of excessive intakes exceeded 90 percent.

SUMMARY AND CONCLUSIONS

This review has identified a number of foods and nutrients for which a notable proportion of children have intake levels inconsistent with recommended intake levels (Table 4-12). During Phase II of this study, the committee will consider these foods and nutrients further and will identify priority foods and nutrients for the Nutrition Standards and Meal Standards of the school meal programs.

TABLE 4-12 Foods and Nutrients Under Consideration in Children's Diets

Age Category	Foods for Which Intakes Are Inadequate, Male and Female	Nutrients for Which Intakes Are Inadequate		Nutrients for Which Intakes Are Excessive[a]	
		Male	Female	Male	Female
Ages 6–8[b]	Fruit Total vegetables Dark green and orange vegetables and legumes Whole grains Total meat and beans Milk	Potassium Fiber	Potassium Fiber	Sodium Saturated fat Total fat Energy[c]	Sodium Saturated fat Total fat Energy[c]
Ages 9–13	Fruit Total vegetables Dark green and orange vegetables and legumes Whole grains Total meat and beans Milk	Magnesium Potassium Vitamins A and E Fiber	Calcium Magnesium Phosphorus Potassium Zinc Vitamins A, C, E Fiber	Sodium Cholesterol Saturated fat	Sodium Energy[c] Total fat Saturated fat
Ages 14–18	Fruit Total vegetables Dark green and orange vegetables and legumes Whole grains Total meat and beans Milk	Magnesium Potassium Vitamins A, C, E Energy[c] Fiber	Calcium Iron Magnesium Phosphorus Potassium Zinc Vitamins A, C, E, B_6, B_{12} Folate Thiamin Energy[c] Fiber	Sodium Cholesterol Saturated fat Total fat	Sodium Cholesterol Saturated fat Total fat

NOTE: Excessive energy intakes for some age-gender groups may not have been identified because of underreporting.

[a]Excessive amounts of discretionary calories were consumed from solid fat and added sugars; this also constitutes concern relative to recommendations to be made by the committee. Usual intakes of added sugars could not be estimated because relevant data were not available in SNDA-III. The committee notes the quantitative amounts of added sugars in Table 4-5. Furthermore, while intakes of *trans* fatty acids also could not be measured, *trans* fatty acids will be considered as appropriate by the committee during Phase II.

[b]Data for children age 5 years were included in the food intake data.

[c]It is difficult to accurately estimate energy intakes because of under- and overreporting of food intake and a lack of accurate information about customary levels of physical activity

5

Proposed Planning Model for Establishing Nutrition Standards for School Meals

The term *planning model* refers to the committee's overall approach and rationale for establishing the Nutrition Standards for the school meal programs. The planning model used to develop the current Nutrition Standards and the related Meal Requirements was based on legislation (USDA, 1995) that provided specifications for the use of the 1995 *Dietary Guidelines for Americans* (HHS/USDA, 1995) and the 1989 Recommended Dietary Allowances (RDAs) (NRC, 1989). Existing law requires that the meals provide one-third and one-fourth of the RDA for lunch and breakfast, respectively, and reflects an approach that was put in place before the development of the Dietary Reference Intakes (DRIs) and guidance on their related applications. In recognition of this, the committee will describe the planned approach to use the DRIs in this Phase I report. The Phase II report will compare differences between basing standards on the RDA approach and basing the standards on the DRI methodology.

The proposed planning method addresses both food and nutrients and incorporates many different factors. Importantly, the method considers that the ultimate goal is to improve children's diets by reducing the apparent prevalence of inadequate and excessive food and nutrient intakes (see criterion 1 in Chapter 3). This chapter considers (1) the setting of nutrient intake targets for school meals, (2) the setting of food intake targets for school meals, and (3) the use of a combined approach of setting both nutrient and food intake targets. This chapter first presents the assumptions that underlie its decision making (see Box 5-1). The setting of nutrient intake targets is covered first because it provides the basis for the content related to food intake targets. For the purposes of this chapter, the term *target* is used in a generic sense and represents a major but preliminary part of the process of setting Nutrition Standards and Meal Requirements for the school meal programs.

BOX 5-1
Assumptions Related to the Proposed Planning Models

General assumptions of the proposed planning model

1. On average, foods offered will be equal to foods consumed; it is inappropriate to inflate the Nutrition Standards or the Menu Requirements, or both, to account for food offered but not consumed.
2. Children with higher or lower energy requirements relative to the Estimated Energy Requirement will adjust their intakes to meet their needs (by altering their intakes at other eating occasions or by eating less of the food served at the school meals).
3. Energy, nutrient, and food intakes can be partitioned into meals.
4. Changes in school meals alone cannot fully eliminate dietary inadequacies. To meet daily goals for food and nutrient intakes, the quality of the non-school foods will also need to improve.

Specific assumptions of the proposed planning model for nutrients

1. The current nutrient intake distributions can be accurately estimated.
2. The assumptions of the EAR cut-point approach are met:
    a. Intake is independent of requirement (assumed true for all nutrients except energy)
    b. The requirement distribution is symmetric (not true for iron)
    c. The variance of intake is greater than the variance of the requirement (assumed to be true for children's intakes)
    d. Observed intake distributions have been adjusted to reflect usual intakes
3. Unless efforts are made to target children in the tails of a nutrient intake distribution, the shape of the distribution will not change if the median intake is changed.

Specific assumptions of the proposed planning model for foods

1. Intakes that adhere to the MyPyramid recommendations will achieve a low prevalence of dietary nutrient inadequacy and a low prevalence of potentially excessive nutrient intakes.
2. On average, the selection of school foods offered within a food group will match the foods that were used to develop the nutrient profiles of the MyPyramid food groups.

SETTING NUTRIENT INTAKE TARGETS FOR SCHOOL MEALS

Background

The DRIs are the current reference values used in the United States and Canada (IOM, 1997, 1998, 2000a, 2001, 2002/2005, 2005). The DRIs replaced the former RDAs (NRC, 1989). As discussed in Institute of Medicine publications concerning applications of the DRIs for the purposes of assessing and planning diets (IOM, 2000b, 2003), the DRIs should now be the basis for assessing and planning the nutrient intakes by population groups, such as schoolchildren.

An appropriate planning model for the derivation of the Nutrition Standards for school meals considers the nutrition needs of the entire population of schoolchildren rather than the needs of specific individuals (IOM, 2003). This approach involves consideration of the distribution of usual intakes when dietary intakes are assessed (as was done in Chapter 4). The planning goal would be to shift this distribution in a more desirable direction (IOM, 2003). The twin goals of planning intakes for groups are to (1) reduce the prevalence of inadequate intakes and (2) reduce the prevalence of intakes at risk of being excessive.

To accomplish these goals in the setting of nutrient intake targets for groups of school children, several types of DRIs may be useful:

- Estimated Energy Requirement (EER),
- Acceptable Macronutrient Distribution Range (AMDR),
- Estimated Average Requirement (EAR),
- Adequate Intake (AI), and
- Tolerable Upper Intake Level (UL).

Values for all of these DRIs for schoolchildren are given in Appendix K.

The RDA, which is also a type of DRI reference value, is not an appropriate target for planning the intakes by population groups because median group intakes at the RDA level are not likely to result in an acceptable prevalence of inadequate intakes within the group (IOM, 2003). See the section *Applying the Dietary Reference Intakes to Reduce the Prevalence of Inadequacy* for more details on the appropriate procedures performed by use of the EAR cut-point method.

Age-Grade Groups for Setting Nutrient Intake Targets

The current age-grade groups specified by the U.S. Department of Agriculture (USDA) for meal programs are shown in Table 5-1.

TABLE 5-1 Current USDA Age-Grade Groups

Groups in National School Lunch Program	Groups in School Breakfast Program
Preschool	Preschool
K[a]–3	K–12
K–6	7–12
4–12	
7–12	

[a]K = kindergarten.
SOURCE: USDA, 2000b, 2008h.

In general, age-grade groups are driven by existing school grade configurations. The age groups used to determine reference values, however, are based on biological and physiological development. Therefore, some of the children in an age-grade group will fall into a different age group for the nutrient reference value. A calculation must be carried out to determine what amount of a nutrient should be assigned as the target for the age-grade groups that correspond to school grade configurations.

During Phase II of this study, the committee will consider the appropriateness of the current age-grade groups, especially in view of the application of DRI values to common school grade configurations. Alternative approaches for various configurations may also be addressed. The committee recognizes that the school grade configurations themselves may change over time and that the configurations may vary among districts. According to the U.S. Department of Education (2000b), a growing number of children attend middle schools, most of which encompass grades 6 through 8, whereas many high schools comprise grades 9 through 12.

For the purposes of illustration relative to the proposed approach described in this Phase I report, however, the committee has used the following grade and age categories. The committee recognizes that the current census data may not support these specific categories:

- Prekindergarten–grade 4: ages 4–8 years
- Grades 5–8: ages 9–13 years
- Grades 9–12: ages 14–18 years

Planning Nutrient Intakes for Heterogeneous

Even when the nutrient needs of schoolchildren are divided according to the age-grade categories listed above, the nutrient needs differ for the children within the two older groups because requirements differ by gender after age 8 years. The DRI age and gender groups are 4–8 years of age for both males and females, ages 9–13 years for males, ages 9–13 years for females, ages 14–18 years for males, and ages 14–18 years for females.

To derive revised calculated Nutrition Standards (see the box in Figure 2-1 in Chapter 2), two approaches have been considered for heterogeneous groups: (1) an approach based the weighted average of the DRI and (2) an approach based on nutrient density.

1. **Weighted average** The current Nutrition Standards for school meals use the weighted average of the RDA for the relevant age-grade group. Calculations based on the RDAs for the ages and genders represented within the school age-grade category are used to obtain the nutrient reference values used for each age-grade category. The weights are determined by using the approximate proportions of the children that fall within each of the reference value age-gender categories. Under this approach, if the new DRIs were used to develop new Nutrition Standards for the illustrative age-grade groups identified earlier, the determinations would be as follows:

- Prekindergarten–grade 4 (ages 4–8 years): the target DRIs for ages 4–8 years would not be weighted because the DRIs apply to both genders.
- Grades 5–8 (ages 9–13 years): the target DRIs would be a weighted average of the reference values for 9- through 13-year-old males and females.
- Grades 9–12 (ages 14–18 years): the target DRIs would be a weighted average of the reference values for 14- through 18-year-old males and females.

2. **Nutrient density** A different approach could be used on the basis of consideration of the nutrient density of the DRI for each of the gender groups within each of the age-grade categories. For each of the gender groups, a target nutrient intake per 1,000 calories would be calculated for each nutrient of interest. The value for the gender with the higher target, expressed as a nutrient density (that is, that value required for the most vulnerable group), would then be used in the process of setting the Nutrition Standards. For example, females may require more nutrients per 1,000 calories because their DRIs are often the same as those for males, but females' calorie intakes are usually lower. If the school meals were designed to provide an amount of a nutrient per 1,000 calories that would meet the needs of most individuals in the more vulnerable group (e.g., females), then the meals would likely meet the nutrient needs of almost everyone in the less vulnerable group (e.g., males). The Nutrition Standards could potentially be higher by this approach than by the weighted-average approach, but the result could be meals that meet the needs of a higher percentage of the students.

With either approach, it is important to examine the projected distribution of daily nutrient intakes around the target DRIs to ensure that very few, if any, would be above the UL, and thus at risk of being excessive (as discussed later in the section, *Applying the Dietary Reference Intakes to Reduce the Prevalence of Intakes at Risk of Being Excessive*). The gender group with the higher energy intake (e.g., males) would be more likely to exceed the UL if the value is the same for males and females.

Applying the Dietary Reference Intakes for Energy

Major decisions to be made by the committee include the determination of calorie levels—in particular, the percentage of the daily calorie intake to be provided by the National School Lunch Program (NSLP) and the School Breakfast Program (SBP) and how this translates to the calories provided in school meals. Consideration of calories is the first step in the committee's proposed plan for setting nutrient intake targets, which is outlined later in this chapter. Elements of the committee's approach to determining calorie levels appear below.

Determining the Calorie Content of School Meals

The EER is the appropriate reference value for use for the planning of energy intakes. Intakes should be planned to meet but not exceed the EER for a DRI age-gender-activity level (IOM, 2003). The average energy requirements determined in the School Nutrition Dietary Assessment Study–III (USDA, 2007a), assuming a low-active level of physical activity, are approximately the following, as explained in Chapter 4:

- Prekindergarten–grade 4 (ages 4–8 years): 1,600 calories/day
- Grades 5–8 (ages 9–13 years): 2,000 calories/day
- Grades 9–12 (ages 14–18 years): 2,400 calories/day

To illustrate the proposed planning approach presented in this Phase I report, the committee used the age-grade groups and calorie levels shown above. Although many children in grade 4 are 9 years of age, the DRI age group for 4–8 years is the age category that is most appropriate for prekindergarten through grade 4. Likewise, the age group of 9–13 years likely covers most configurations for the children in middle schools. However, given the variability of calorie needs within these categories, during Phase II the committee will also consider specifying a range of energy intakes within these age-grade categories.

To gain perspective on the current calorie standards, the committee estimated the extent to which the current standard for the calorie content of school lunches (see Appendix H) contributes to children's estimated requirements for calories. Because the school lunch is required to provide one-third (approximately 33 percent) of the day's calorie intake, the committee estimated a full-day's intake by multiplying the current standard for age-grade groups by three. For the kindergarten through grade 3 group (ages 5–8 years), for example, the calculation and comparison are as follows:

Current meal standard	633 calories/lunch meal
Multiplier (based on a lunch providing one-third of the energy requirement for the day)	×3
Calculated daily energy intake	1,899 calories/day
Average daily energy requirement for age-grade group	1,600 calories/day
Current meal standard as a percentage of the average daily energy requirement for the age-grade group	40%

Thus, the current energy standard for the lunch meal provides about 40 percent of the day's energy needs for this group, rather than 33 percent. Stated differently, for the youngest age group, the calculated daily amount is almost 300 calories per day higher than the average amount of energy required for children ages 4–8 years. Comparable calculations for the other age-grade groups show that the current energy standards for the lunch meal also substantially exceed one-third of the estimated daily requirement for calories.

Determining the Percentage of Calorie Intake to Be Supplied by School Meals

By law, the current school meals must supply, on average and at a minimum, one-third of the day's energy requirements in a school lunch and one-fourth in a school breakfast. The School Nutrition and Dietary Assessment Study-III found that the school lunch typically supplies approximately 30 percent of the day's energy intake for schoolchildren, whereas the school breakfast supplies approximately 20 percent of the day's energy intake (USDA, 2007a). For the purposes of this Phase I report, the committee used 30 percent and 20 percent of intake as the amounts of energy to be supplied by school lunch and school breakfast, respectively. During Phase II, however, the committee will examine other sources (such as the National Health and Nutrition Examination Survey) that provide data on typical calorie intakes at lunch and breakfast as a percentage of the total day's intake to determine the percentage of calorie intake to be supplied by school meals. It appears possible that the use of percentages that are lower than the current calorie standards may be more realistic for planning purposes for lunch and breakfast, especially in view of the observation that many children snack throughout the day. The use of lower percentages might also be less likely to contribute to the overconsumption of energy than the use of the current percentages prescribed by law.

Applying the Dietary Reference Intakes for Macronutrient Ranges

The AMDRs specify the desirable ranges of macronutrient intakes as a percentage of energy intake. AMDRs for schoolchildren have been set for five macronutrients: total fat, linoleic acid, alpha-linolenic acid, carbohydrate, and protein. The desirable ranges of values are given in Appendix K. Ideally, the amounts of macronutrients provided in school meals should minimize intakes that fall outside these ranges.

Applying the Dietary Reference Intakes to Reduce the Prevalence of Inadequacy

Nutrients with an Estimated Average Requirement

For most nutrients for which an EAR is used, the current prevalence of nutrient inadequacy may be estimated by the EAR cut-point method (see Chapter 4). If the prevalence of inadequacy is too high, then one goal of the planning process is to reduce the prevalence of inadequacy to an acceptable level. For the purposes of this Phase I report, a 5 percent prevalence of inadequacy is used as an example. The committee may consider other levels, based on the feasibility of implementation and other relevant factors. Furthermore, if some children's eating patterns differ substantially from those of the majority of their peers, then other approaches may be needed to reach children at the lower end of the intake distributions. Finally, the cost of providing the extra amounts of nutrients, which may be revealed through the committee's future analyses, may influence the committee's recommendations for some nutrients.

One assumption that could be made in developing recommendations for revisions to the Nutrition Standards is that any changes in the school meals will be directly reflected in the total daily intake. If this assumption is correct, then alteration of the nutrient content of the school meals would shift the distribution of usual nutrient intakes without changing the shape of the distribution. Under this assumption, it is possible to calculate how far the distribution needs to be moved (IOM, 2003), as follows:

- If the goal is to have 5 percent of usual intakes below the EAR, then the 5th percentile of the intake distribution should be positioned at the EAR.
- If the shape of the distribution does not change, then each point on the distribution, including the median, would change by the same amount.
- The new median of the distribution could be calculated as the old median plus the amount of the change.
- The new median would be considered the target median intake (TMI) and could be used as the basis for the establishment of Nutrition Standards for school meals.

For example, assume that the EAR for a hypothetical nutrient is 10 milligrams (mg) per day and that 30 percent of the group has usual intakes below the EAR. To reduce the estimated prevalence of inadequacy from 30 percent to 5 percent, it would be necessary to increase the intake at the 5th percentile to 10 mg/day. If the intake at the 5th percentile was currently 4 mg/day, for example, then the distribution would need to be shifted by +7 mg/day (Figure 5-1). If the intake median (the intake at the 50th percentile) was currently 26 mg/day, then the TMI would be 33 mg/day.

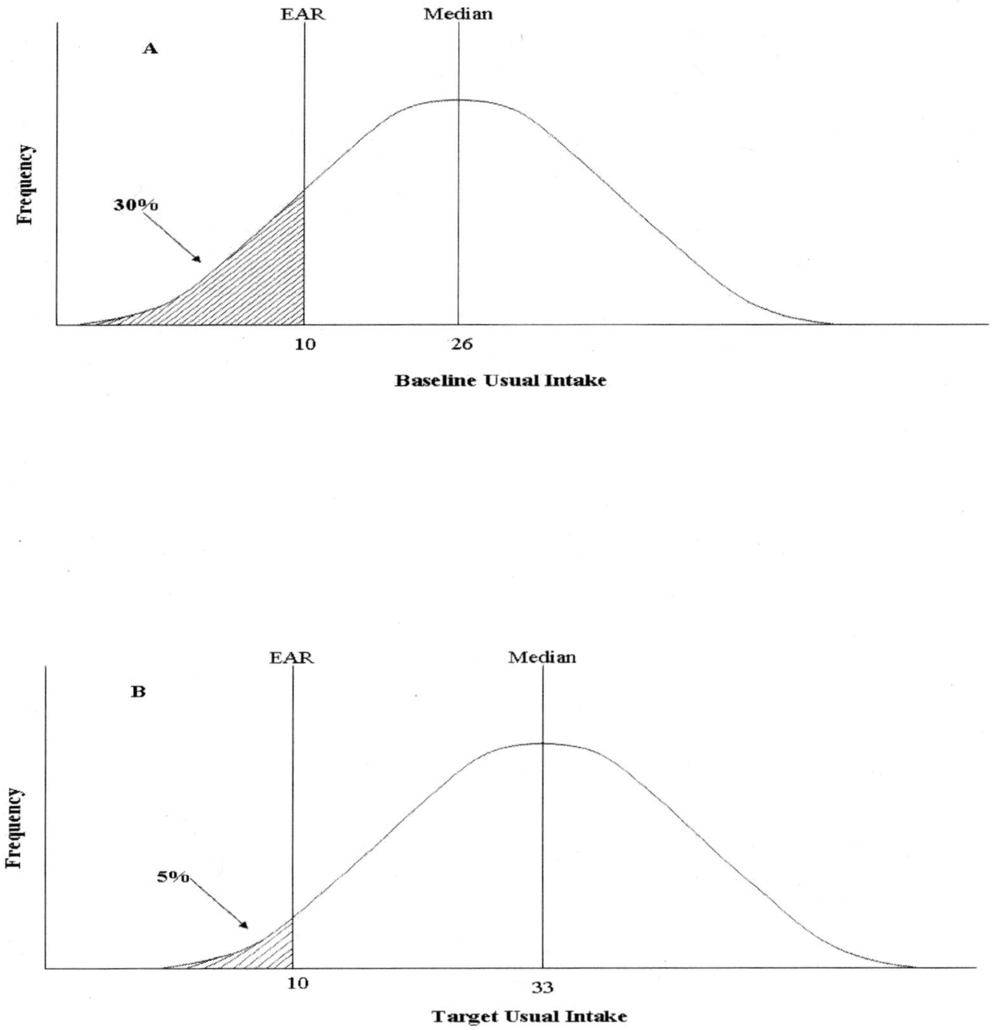

FIGURE 5-1 Concept of setting a TMI. (A) Baseline usual nutrient intake distribution, in which the prevalence of inadequate intake (percentage below the EAR) is about 30 percent. Shifting the baseline distribution up so that the prevalence of inadequate intakes reflects the planning goal (in this example, 5 percent below the EAR) attains the target usual nutrient intake distribution around the median (the TMI) (B).
SOURCE: Adapted from IOM, 2006b.

By using data from the School Nutrition and Dietary Assessment Study-III study on the distribution of schoolchildren's usual intakes, a TMI can be calculated for the nutrients of interest in schoolchildren's diets. As an example, Table 5-2 presents the median intakes of selected nutrients reported by children ages 14–18 years and compares the TMIs associated with a 5 percent prevalence of inadequacy to those median intakes. Vitamin E is an example of a nutrient for which the proposed TMI would be much higher than the current median intake. As a result, the target may need to be revised because of concerns about feasibility and acceptability. Table 5-2 also presents TMIs for nutrients that do not have an EAR. For a discussion of how those TMIs were set, see the next section, *Nutrients with an Adequate Intake*.

TABLE 5-2 Basis for TMI Values for Children Ages 14–18 Years, Selected Nutrients

Nutrient	Reported Median Intake	5th Percentile of Current Intake Distribution	EAR[a]	TMI[b]
Protein (g/kg/d)	1.3	0.8	0.72	1.22[c]
Vitamin A (μg RAE/d)	580	243	558	895
Vitamin E (mg αT/d)	6.5	3.9	12	14.6
Vitamin C (mg/d)	76	26	60	110
Thiamin (mg/d)	1.7	0.9	1.0	1.8
Riboflavin (mg/d)	2.3	1.2	1.0	2.1
Niacin (mg/d)	22.9	13.8	11.5	20.6
Vitamin B_6 (mg/d)	1.8	1.0	1.1	1.9
Folate (μg DFE/d)	550	284	330	596
Vitamin B_{12} (μg /d)	5.2	2.4	2.0	4.8
Calcium (mg/d)	1,073	510	N/A	1,300
Phosphorus (mg/d)	1,440	823	1,055	1,672
Magnesium (mg/d)	258	156	320	422
Iron (mg/d)	15.3	8.7	7.8	N/C[d]
Zinc (mg/d)	12.2	6.8	7.9	13.3
Sodium (mg/d)	3,677	2,361	N/A	2,300[e]
Potassium (mg/d)	2,625	1,622	N/A	4,700
Fiber (g/d)	13.9	7.8	N/A	32

NOTE: αT = α-tocopheral; d = day; DFE = dietary folate equivalents; g = gram; mg = milligram; N/A = not applicable because an AI rather than an EAR has been set for these nutrients; N/C = not calculated; RAE = retinol activity equivalents; μg = microgram.

[a]Average EAR of males and females (IOM, 2006b).

[b]TMI is defined as the median of the target usual intake distribution; for illustrative purposes, the TMIs shown here are calculated as reported median intake + (EAR – intake at 5th percentile); for nutrients with an AI, the TMI is equal to the AI; all TMIs are the average for males and females.

[c]Approximately 74 g/d for a boy weighing 61 kg and 66 g/d for a girl weighing 54 kg.

[d]A TMI for iron cannot be calculated by the EAR cut-point method because iron requirements are not symmetrically distributed.

[e]To foster palatability, and for consistency with the 2005 *Dietary Guidelines for Americans*, the UL is used as the TMI for sodium.

SOURCE: USDA, 2007a.

Although an EAR has been set for iron, a TMI for iron is not included in Table 5-2. The EAR cut-point method cannot be used for iron because the distribution of the requirement is not symmetric. The prevalence of inadequacy must be estimated from probability tables (IOM, 2001), and this may be done during Phase II of the study. Otherwise, the same approach as described above may be used to calculate the TMI for iron. Because intake at the 5th percentile (8.7 mg/day) approximates the EAR (7.8 mg/day) in the example shown in Table 5-2, it is likely that the TMI would be close to the current median intake (15.3 mg/day).

Nutrients with an Adequate Intake

An AI rather than an EAR is used for some nutrients. For these nutrients, a prevalence of inadequacy cannot be determined. If the median of the usual intake distribution is equal to the AI, however, a low prevalence of inadequacy can be assumed. Thus, for nutrients with an AI, the TMI can be set equal to the AI (as shown for potassium and fiber in Table 5-2). Although an AI has been set for sodium, the committee proposes to use a higher value (the UL) as the TMI. The higher value would be more consistent with the acceptability of the school meals to students. The use of the UL is consistent with the 2005 *Dietary Guidelines for Americans*. For sodium, the goal would be to reduce the median intake to the TMI.

The derivation of the AI differs substantially for different nutrients and for different age-gender groups. Nonetheless, for nutrients with an AI, the AI is still the most appropriate target to use for the planning of school meals. For the AIs that were not set specifically on the basis of the current intakes by a healthy population, however, it is possible that median usual intakes at the AI level will not always be associated with a low prevalence of inadequate intakes.

Potential Applications of Target Mean Intakes

As shown in Table 5-2 for schoolchildren ages 14–18 years, the median usual intakes of some nutrients exceed the estimated TMI and the median usual intakes of many nutrients are well below the estimated TMI. Children in the younger age groups have more favorable intakes of many nutrients. For children ages 6–8 years, for example, the median usual intakes of 13 nutrients[1] exceed the estimated TMI (data not shown). Thus, if the revised Nutrition Standards for school meals are based on a TMI, the resulting daily intakes are likely to be below the current usual intakes for several nutrients, especially for the younger age groups.

Because school meals are not intended to provide 100 percent of the daily nutrient intake, it is reasonable to set the Nutrition Standards on the basis of a percentage of the TMI. For example, the Nutrition Standard for a nutrient might be 20 percent of the nutrient's TMI for breakfast and 30 percent for lunch. The percentage of a nutrient's TMI that is used as the school meal target may vary across the nutrients. For example, the percentage goals for nutrients in the inadequate intake column of Table 4-12 in Chapter 4 might be higher than for those whose daily reported intakes are adequate. However, it is unlikely that school meals can fully compensate for all nutrient inadequacies. Thus, improvements in dietary intake at other eating occasions will be necessary to meet all of the daily intake goals.

---

[1]These nutrients exclude sodium.

Applying the Dietary Reference Intakes to Reduce the Prevalence of Intakes at Risk of Being Excessive

The UL should be used to evaluate whether planned meals are likely to result in a risk of excessive intakes. Ideally, the predicted prevalence of intakes above the UL should be close to zero for all age-gender groups. If the prevalence of intakes above the UL is not low, it may be necessary to adjust the target nutrient intake distribution so that the prevalence of inadequacy and the prevalence of intakes above the UL are acceptably balanced. For some intake distributions, it may be desirable to investigate ways to change the shape of the nutrient intake distribution, rather than trying to move the current distribution up or down. There may be nutrients for which it would be desirable to reduce the prevalence of very high or very low intakes, without changing intakes in the middle of the distribution. For example, if highly fortified foods are contributing to very high nutrient intakes for a few individuals, these foods might be removed from the menu. Likewise, if some children avoid foods (such as milk) that are rich sources of certain nutrients, then including acceptable substitutes in the menu might increase their intakes of those nutrients. However, detailed examinations of the impact of interventions (such as feeding programs) on the shape of an intake distribution are almost nonexistent (IOM, 2003, p. 88).

Proposed Method for Setting Nutrient Intake Targets for School Meals

On the basis of earlier guidance from the Institute of Medicine (IOM, 2003), the committee has proposed the following seven steps for the setting of nutrient intake targets for school meals.

1. For each age-gender group, determine the target daily energy intake and the goals for the percentages of energy to be provided by breakfast and lunch.
2. For nutrients with an EAR:
    a. Determine the acceptable prevalence of inadequacy and the acceptable prevalence of excessive intakes.
    b. Determine a target nutrient intake distribution to achieve these goals. The median of this distribution is the TMI for the age-gender group.
    c. If necessary, adjust the target nutrient intake distribution so that the prevalence of inadequacy and the prevalence of intakes above the UL are acceptably balanced.
3. For nutrients (other than sodium) with an AI:
    a. Set the TMI equal to the AI for the age-gender group.
    b. If necessary, adjust the TMI to reduce the prevalence of intakes above the UL.
4. For sodium, set the TMI equal to the UL for the age-gender group.
5. For each nutrient, apply the age-gender TMIs to develop a TMI for each grade category using either a weighted average or a nutrient-density approach.
6. For each nutrient, determine the goal for the percentage of a day's intake to be provided by school breakfast and school lunch, and apply the percentage to the TMI to obtain the school meal target.
7. Evaluate the proposed school meal targets in terms of feasibility, cost, and acceptability. Revise the targets as needed to provide an acceptable balance of adequacy, avoidance of excess, feasibility, cost, and acceptability. Sodium is an example of a nutrient for which the proposed TMI may need to be revised because of concerns about feasibility and acceptability.

The resulting nutrient intake targets would be consistent with the goals of planning school meals to reduce the prevalence of inadequacy and to reduce the risk of excessive intakes among schoolchildren. However, the impact of changes in the Nutrition Standards and Meal Requirements on children's daily intakes cannot be completely predicted. An intake assessment performed after changes are implemented by USDA would be needed to determine the impact.

SETTING FOOD INTAKE TARGETS FOR SCHOOL MEALS

Background

To develop food intake targets that are based on the current *Dietary Guidelines for Americans* (at present, the year 2005 edition), the committee proposes to incorporate the MyPyramid food intake patterns as shown in Appendix J. The use of food intake targets that are consistent with the MyPyramid food intake patterns would be consistent with adherence to the *Dietary Guidelines for Americans*. As described in Chapter 4, the committee used MyPyramid to assess food intakes for children ages 4–8 years, 9–13 years, and 14–18 years.

MyPyramid was designed by using the most recent RDAs or AIs for 17 micronutrients and fiber and the AMDRs (Britten et al., 2006). In the development of MyPyramid, the nutrient profiles of each of the food groups were used to ensure that the specified number of servings from the MyPyramid food groups would meet those nutrient intake targets (Marcoe et al., 2006).

Comparison of Food and Nutrient Intake Targets

Because the RDAs are not an appropriate target for use for the planning of the intakes by groups (IOM, 2003), the committee used a new approach to investigate the applicability of basing food intake targets on MyPyramid. In particular, the committee compared the amount of nutrients provided by MyPyramid intake patterns to TMIs, which, as described above, would reduce the predicted prevalence of nutrient inadequacy to an acceptable level. Table 5-3 makes this comparison by using the TMIs from Table 5-2. For children ages 14–18 years, the amount of nutrients provided by the 2,400-calorie MyPyramid food intake pattern would exceed the TMI for all but two nutrients (vitamin E and potassium), and all nutrients would be provided at 73 percent or more of the respective TMIs (see the rightmost column of Table 5-3). For the children ages 6–8 years, the amount of nutrients provided by the MyPyramid intake patterns would exceed the TMI for all nutrients except vitamin E and potassium (data not shown). For children ages 9–13 years, vitamin E, which would be provided at only 73 percent, was the only nutrient that would not exceed the TMI (data not shown).

TABLE 5-3 Contents of Selected Nutrients for a 2,400-Calorie MyPyramid Food Intake Pattern, Absolute Value and Percentage of the TMI

Nutrient	Nutrient content of MyPyramid food intake pattern for 2,400 calories/day	MyPyramid Nutrients as % of TMI[a]
Protein (g/d)	105	128[b]
Vitamin A (μg RAE/d)	1,126	126
Vitamin E (mg αT/d)	10.7	73
Vitamin C (mg/d)	163	148
Thiamin (mg/d)	2.4	133
Riboflavin (mg/d)	3.1	148
Niacin (mg/d)	27.3	133
Vitamin B_6 (mg/d)	2.9	153
Folate (μg DFE/d)	822	138
Vitamin B_{12} (μg/d)	9.2	192
Calcium (mg/d)	1,388	107
Phosphorus (mg/d)	1,961	117
Magnesium (mg/d)	440	104
Iron (mg/d)	21.5	141[c]
Zinc (mg/d)	16.7	126
Sodium (mg/d)	2,136	142
Potassium (mg/d)	4,523	96
Fiber (g/d)	37	116

NOTE: αT = α-tocopheral; d = day; DFE = dietary folate equivalents; g = gram; mg = milligram; RAE = retinol activity equivalents; μg = microgram.

[a]TMIs are based on the values in the last column of Table 5-2.

[b]Based on an average weight of 67 kg (reference weight for an 18 year-old male (IOM, 2002/2005, p. 137))—the age and gender with the highest TMI within this age group.

[c]For illustrative purposes, this assumes that the iron TMI is equal to the current median intake of 15.3 mg/day.

SOURCE: Britten et al., 2006. Reprinted from the Journal of Nutrition Education and Behavior, Volume 38, P. Britten, K. Marcoe, S. Yamini, and C. Davis, Development of Food Intake Patterns for the MyPyramid Food Guidance System, pages S78–S92, Copyright (2006), with permission from Elsevier.

Comparison of MyPyramid Intake Patterns with Current School Meal Requirements

To compare the amounts of food specified by the MyPyramid food intake pattern with the current school meal requirements for a school lunch, the committee divided the total daily MyPyramid amounts for selected calorie levels by three. (By law, school lunch must provide one-third of a day's intake of calories and nutrients.) Based on the committee's calculations, the amount of food recommended in the MyPyramid food intake patterns exceeds the current minimum amounts required for the majority of food groups in NSLP meal patterns. A table illustrating the MyPyramid food amounts for 800 calories (2,400 calories/3, the calorie level that might apply to school lunches for children ages 14–18 years) is located in Appendix L. For comparison, Appendix L also shows the current minimum food group amounts for both a traditional and an enhanced meal in the NSLP for children in grades 7–12 and the percentage of the MyPyramid food intake pattern amount represented.

By quantity, the primary difference is for total fruits and vegetables. The amount of fruits and vegetables in the current Meal Requirements for a traditional lunch is less than half the MyPyramid amount of approximately 1.67 cup equivalents. Similar differences are seen for the other two age-grade categories. MyPyramid is very specific about the quality of the foods within the food groups. For example, MyPyramid provides targets for fruits and vegetables separately, and it specifies separate targets for five vegetable subgroups: dark green vegetables, orange vegetables, legumes, starchy vegetables, and other vegetables. MyPyramid also specifies that half of the grain intake should be whole grain. Such specifications are not currently included in the NSLP Meal Requirements.

Importantly, MyPyramid assumes that all foods are provided in their lowest-fat form and have no added sugars. Unlike the current Meal Requirements, MyPyramid includes a value for discretionary calories, which are calories from any source that can be used flexibly (these calories are often from added sugars or solid fats or fat from foods that are not in their lowest-fat form, such as milk with 2 percent fat). However, if the MyPyramid meal plans are followed, few discretionary calorie are available: for a lunch meal that is one-third of the daily calories, the discretionary calorie levels would be 44 calories/meal for the 1,600-calorie/day plan, 89 calories/meal for the 2,000-calorie/day plan, and 121 calories/meal for the 2,400-calorie/day plan.

Proposed Method for Setting Food Intake Targets for School Meals

The following three steps outline a potentially useful general approach to applying current dietary guidance to the planning of school meals:

1. Select appropriate energy levels.
2. Apply the goal for the percentage of the day's intake (e.g., 20 and 30 percent for breakfast and lunch, respectively) to the MyPyramid food intake pattern for the energy level (by using the amounts in the MyPyramid food groups shown in Appendix J, Table J-2) to obtain amounts of each food group to recommend. For some food groups, amounts may be specified per week rather than per day, to achieve practical portion sizes.
3. Consider the recommendations for discretionary calories. Staying within these recommendations may require greatly decreasing or eliminating the use of foods that are high in fats and added sugars.

SUMMARY: COMBINING THE NUTRIENT INTAKE AND FOOD INTAKE TARGETS

Although the committee recognizes the need for nutrient intake targets, the process for setting nutrient intake targets described in this chapter involves many assumptions. Thus, there are many uncertainties about the accuracy of the estimated TMIs. A comparison of the TMIs with the nutrients provided by the MyPyramid food intake patterns shows that adherence to MyPyramid results in diets whose nutrient contents almost always meet or exceed the TMIs. Moreover, adherence to MyPyramid results in diets that are consistent with the *Dietary Guidelines for Americans*. To achieve the planning objectives, the committee will consider recommending that food targets be emphasized in the development of the Nutrition Standards and Meal Requirements for school meals. In particular, the committee may begin by using the MyPyramid food plans as the basis for the school meal targets and then assess projected nutrient intake distributions (using information about the shape of current intake distributions) to determine if the desired objectives are likely to be achieved. As with any method of planning school meals, it would be necessary to assess the children's actual nutrient intakes after changes are implemented by USDA to determine if the planning objectives have been achieved.

The school meal food targets would be supplemented with selected school meal nutrient targets for nutrients such as sodium, total fat, saturated fat, cholesterol, and a target for added sugars. An iterative process will be used to find the most satisfactory balance of food group targets to achieve consistency with *Dietary Guidelines for Americans* and DRIs. If it is workable, this approach may offer an additional advantage: the simplification of meal planning and monitoring.

6

Proposed Phase II Analyses: Sensitivity Analysis, Cost Implications, and Market Effects

The development of sound recommendations for revised Nutrition Standards and Meal Requirements will require extensive analyses. It is likely that the results of the analyses will point to the need to make adjustments to initial proposals for revisions. In developing its final recommendations, the committee will balance the findings from the analyses to achieve a reliable correspondence with the criteria presented in Chapter 3 of this report. The following sections provide an overview of the proposed sensitivity analysis, a specific description of the methods proposed for analysis of cost implications, and a description of how market effects will be estimated.

SENSITIVITY ANALYSIS

In the process of carrying out its tasks during Phase II, the committee will compare the recommended revisions to the Nutrition Standards and Meal Requirements with the current standards for the School Breakfast Program (SBP) and the National School Lunch Program (NSLP). The sensitivity analysis will critically examine each recommendation with respect to likely benefits and consequences. Specifically, the committee will examine the following factors:

1. food intake sample menus with respect to improved adherence to the *2005 Dietary Guidelines for Americans* (HHS/USDA, 2005),
2. possible effects of nutrient intake contributions from school meals with respect to the prevalence of inadequacy and excessive intake as defined by the Dietary Reference Intakes, (DRIs),
3. cost and administrative impacts on food service operations,
4. menu characteristics that influence acceptance by the students, and
5. participation rates.

One method of examining nutrient intake with respect to the prevalence of inadequacy and excessive intake as defined by the DRIs will be to take the mean nutrient content of the recommended food group intakes (across the day), and determine what the prevalence of inadequacy and excess would be using the shape of the current nutrient intake distribution. This method might be particularly useful in estimating whether intakes would exceed the Tolerable Upper Intake Levels. Assumptions about the levels of acceptance of the proposed changes by students, participation rates, and the degree of supplementation or substitution resulting from the recommendations will be considered by using a range of values. For many changes, the likely benefits and consequences will be multidimensional, in the sense that several of the key factors will be affected by the recommended revisions. For example, a likely consequence of eliminating flavored milk (i.e., chocolate or strawberry) would be to reduce the intake of added sugars, as recommended by the *Dietary Guidelines for Americans*. However, another likely consequence would be to reduce the consumption of milk and thus reduce calcium intakes, thereby increasing the likelihood of inadequate calcium intakes. Similarly, a change designed to reduce the prevalence of inadequate intakes might be so unattractive to students that the net effect of the change would be the opposite of what was intended. During Phase II, the committee will review publications that provided data on menu characteristics and other factors that influence meal acceptance by students. The committee will examine the recommendations relative to each of the factors separately and consider qualitatively the net effect of the combined benefits and consequences.

The sensitivity analysis will rely on published studies and reports, when they are available, as well as the experiences of practitioners in the school food service industry. A key type of information will be the experiences of school districts that have implemented changes similar to those recommended in the proposed standards. Whenever possible, the sensitivity of the likely benefits and consequences will be assessed with respect to the uncertainties in the assumptions used to evaluate the recommendations.

ADDRESSING COST IMPLICATIONS

Because the U.S. Department of Agriculture (USDA) does not anticipate that additional funding will be available to schools to implement the revised requirements, any proposed revisions to the Nutrition Standards and Meal Requirements used for the school meal programs should be examined with respect to how change may be affected and increases in costs may be minimized. The committee's intent is to design recommended revisions that will keep program costs economical and as close as possible to current levels (adjusted for inflation). The objective of maintaining program costs at current levels is particularly challenging during periods of rapidly rising food costs and other costs, as was the case in 2008. This section provides an overview of the committee's proposed approach and the data sources that it will consider when it estimates the anticipated economic impacts of its recommendations. Use of this approach will allow consideration of the implications of the recommended changes for school food authorities (SFAs) and commodity markets under the assumptions of full substitution and full supplementation (defined below) and the impacts at the expected levels of substitution and supplementation.

> *Substitution* may involve either the addition or the deletion of a food outside of the school meal: (1) if a food is deleted from the school meal, the students replace it in their diet by obtaining the food elsewhere and eating it, or (2) if a food is added to the school meal, the student drops it from foods ordinarily eaten outside of the school meal.

Supplementation occurs if the students and the members of their households do not make any changes in food expenditures or food consumption outside of the changes in the foods consumed in the school meal.

The key sources of information for this task will be published national-level studies of meal and food costs (USDA, 1998b, 2008e) and information based on the experiences of school districts that have implemented these or similar changes.

Background

The fiscal year 2007 total costs for the SBP and the NSLP were estimated to be $2.2 billion and $8.7 billion, respectively (USDA/ERS, 2008). Most of the support from the USDA to participating school districts, independent schools, and institutions is in the form of a cash reimbursement for each meal served. As described in Table 2-4 of Chapter 2, the basic cash reimbursement rates are calculated annually and are published in the *Federal Register* each July for immediate application to school financial claims submitted for the new school year (July through June of the next school year).

Higher reimbursement rates are available to schools with high percentages of low-income students and to schools that are determined to be in severe need because they serve a high percentage of children eligible for free and reduced-price meals (see the bottom part of Table 2-4). Schools also are entitled by law to receive commodity foods at a value of $0.2075 for each lunch meal served during the previous school year. When market conditions dictate, bonus commodities may be available to schools. In the 1996–1997 school year, the most recent complete set of data available, school districts acquired 83 percent of the value of all food as purchased food, 4 percent as processed foods containing donated commodities, and 13 percent as donated commodities[1] (USDA, 1998b). Milk and other dairy products accounted for almost one-fourth of the total value of the foods acquired; and bakery products, red meats, poultry, fruits and fruit juices, vegetables, and prepared foods each accounted for about 10 percent of the total value of the foods acquired. Commodities accounted for the majority of the total value of some products, including turkey products, beef products, cheese, flour, and eggs (USDA, 1998b). However, the composition of USDA commodity donations varies from year to year (USDA, 2008b).

Since 1996, the cost of food has increased substantially. In the 12 years between May 1996 and May 2008, the cost of food away from home expenditures increased by nearly 41 percent, and the cost increased 4.3 percent between May[2] 2006 and May 2007. The prices of dairy and related products, eggs, and processed fruits and vegetables rose at a faster rate than those of many other food items between May 2006 and May 2008 (Table 6-1). The increase in the prices of other product (such as meats) was less than the average increase. Thus, today, school districts must make significant adjustments to accommodate rising costs.

---

[1]A 2008 report now indicates that approximately 20 percent of food served in school lunches is derived from commodities (CFPA, 2008).

[2]May is the month of adjustment for the school meal programs.

TABLE 6-1 Percent Change in the Consumer Price Index for Food for All Urban Consumers (May)

	Percent Change	
Item	2006–2007	2007–2008
All foods	3.9	5.1
Food at home	4.4	5.8
Food away from home	3.3	4.3
Bakery products	4.6	11.1
Dairy and related products	3.5	11.0
Fluid milk	7.5	10.2
Eggs	29.6	18.2
Meat	4.7	0.53
Fruit and vegetables	6.7	4.4
Fresh	7.7	3.3
Processed	2.9	8.4

NOTE: The adjusted increase for the school meal programs was 4.272 percent in the 2007–2008 school year. This percent change differs from the number for food away from home reported here (4.256 percent) because of rounding.
SOURCE: U.S. Bureau of Labor Statistics, 2008.

Cost of Food to School Food Authorities

Food purchasing practices are complex, and in turn, so are the costs and the sources of foods acquired. Table 1-3 in Chapter 1 provides brief summaries of relevant findings from cost studies and a school food purchasing study, along with the websites that can be accessed to obtain further information.

Procurement and purchasing regulations are determined at the federal level, however states policies vary considerably from state to state. Some states (for example, Minnesota) allow districts to purchase food with other districts under what is known as a joint powers agreement. Such agreements allow school districts to increase their purchasing powers. Nevertheless, SFAs' food costs vary widely for a variety of reasons, including the following:

- the methods that the state uses to handle commodities (as well as the values of commodities that a school district receives, which depends on participation the previous year);
- the purchasing rules of the state or district;
- geographical differences that govern the availability of fresh produce, dairy products, and grain products;
- bid pricing and purchasing power;
- distributor costs and district and distributor locations;
- the school's location in a metropolitan or a rural area;
- student, geographical, or cultural food preferences; and
- the variety of cooking and food production methods used (for example, the use of an onsite versus a central kitchen with satellite sites and convenience heat-and-serve food preparation versus from cooking from scratch).

School districts do have the flexibility to change menus as needed, depending on market prices, the availability of certain products, and other factors. Nevertheless the menu must still meet the Meal Requirements. When a major beef recall occurred in spring 2008, for example, districts (SFAs) had to substitute chicken or turkey. The substitutions resulted in some cost variations and in problems with meeting the Meal Requirement for iron.

USDA manages the procurement of agricultural (food) commodities through the Agricultural Marketing Service (AMS) and the Kansas City Commodity Office of the Farm Service Agency. AMS purchases a variety of food products designed to stabilize the prices in agricultural commodity markets. The fresh and processed foods customarily purchased under these programs include fruit and vegetables, beef and pork, poultry and egg products, and fish. The Kansas City office purchases grain products, including pasta, processed cereal, flours, crackers, ready-to-eat cereals, rice products, corn products, and miscellaneous dairy products; the Kansas City office also facilitates food distribution and multifood warehouse contracts.

Benchmark for Estimated School Meal Costs

To derive a benchmark for estimated school meal costs, the committee considered the following data from a national survey of SFAs for the 2005–2006 school year (USDA, 2008e):

- The costs reported to be required to run the NSLP and the SBP, which include
    - food costs (about 46 percent),
    - labor costs (slightly less than 45 percent), and
    - other costs (supplies, contract services, and indirect charges incurred by school districts, slightly less than 10 percent).

School districts also incur costs in support of SFA operations that are not charged to the SFA (unreported costs not charged to the food service budget or transfers of local educational money to cover food service budget losses in excess of the program fund balance).

- For the average SFA, the national mean reported costs of producing a reimbursable lunch and a reimbursable breakfast and the mean cost of the NSLP and the SBP meals are shown in Table 6-2. Table 6-2 does not provide data on the variability of meal costs, which may be substantial during a school year or even during a single week.

TABLE 6-2 Comparison of the Reported Costs of Producing a Reimbursable Meal, NSLP and SBP, by Unit of Analysis, 2005–2006 School Year

	NSLP		SBP	
Type of Cost	Mean SFA Cost	Mean Meal Cost	Mean SFA Cost	Mean Meal Cost
Reported[a]	$2.36	$2.28	$1.92	$1.46
Food	$1.09	$0.98	$0.73	$0.65
Labor	$1.05	$1.04	$1.02	$0.64
Other	$0.23	$0.25	$0.17	$0.17

[a]Reported costs may not equal the sum of the component costs because of rounding.
SOURCE: USDA, 2008e.

By the use of either unit of analysis (the mean SFA cost or the mean meal cost), food and labor costs represented most (approximately 90 percent) of the average reported costs. The full costs of meals, which include the costs incurred but not charged to the SFA, are higher than the mean SFA and mean meal cost for both lunch and breakfast.

The food costs and the associated reported labor and administrative costs shown in Table 6-2 provide a benchmark for estimated school meal costs. In addition, the committee will consider indirect costs for labor, equipment, and other items that may not be reported. These indirect costs have also been investigated (USDA, 2008e) and used to determine the total costs of the meals.

Although these costs are reported on the basis of average meal costs, it is useful to note that ultimately, SFAs establish costs and resolve the reimbursement process at the end of a menu cycle and at the end of the school year. Hence, for planning purposes, there may be considerable variability in costs on a specific day.

Proposed Method of Assigning Costs and Changes in Costs for a Set of Representative School Menus

Use of a Representative Set of Menus

Assessment of the impacts of reimbursable lunch and reimbursable breakfast meals on costs requires data on the relative amounts of foods used in a representative (typical or average) meal and the relative prices of the individual food items used. During Phase II, the committee proposes to

1. select a representative set of menus for the lunch and breakfast meals by drawing from menus for each type of meal from frequently observed menus (and food items) from data for elementary schools from the School Nutrition Dietary Assessment Study-III (SNDA-III);
2. estimate the cost of the representative menu set; and
3. use the representative menu set to examine the cost implications of offering that menu versus a set of menus planned by using proposed revisions to the Nutrition Standards and Meal Requirements. For the purposes of the cost analysis, the committee will use a menu plan for an elementary school and include 5 days of menus in the representative week.

To test possible changes in cost resulting from changes to the representative menu set (substitutions of foods, addition or deletion of foods, or respecification of products), the committee will use a method similar to that described below for the determination of baseline cost data.

Determination of Baseline Cost Data

Baseline cost data that use available nationally representative food cost data at the individual food item level will be developed, and the costs will be adjusted to current (2005–2006 school year or more current) costs by following these steps:

- Use the most recent cost data at the individual food item level, namely, the data from the 1996–1997 school year (USDA, 1998b).[3]

[3]The more recent Cost Study II (USDA, 2008e) cannot be used for this purpose because it includes no data on specific food items.

- Adjust the aggregate week's meal costs to the more current period (the 2005–2006 school year or later) by using the Consumer Price Index for Food Away from Home (CPI-FAFH) (U.S. Bureau of Labor Statistics, 2008) to adjust the data for inflation.
- Evaluate the adjusted food and average meal cost data.
- Calibrate the data, if necessary, to more recent estimates of meal costs available from a study of the Food and Nutrition Service of USDA (USDA, 2008e).

Although this approach is limited in its ability to ensure that the total cost of all meals adds up to the total value of the food acquisitions and other costs for the school meal program, it is useful for estimating the cost implications of possible adjustments in the types and amounts of foods needed to meet the recommended revisions to the Nutrition Standards.

Test Application of the Determination of Base Food Cost

To explore the feasibility of determining base food costs of a meal for a representative menu, the committee applied the method described above to a sample 5-day week of lunch menus for an elementary school, as shown in Appendix M and described in the three steps below. The lunch menus were selected from the most commonly used school menus reported in SNDA-III (and compiled by Abt Associates for the committee's use).

1. The food items for School 1 were matched to food item codes and assigned the cost from the 1996–1997 school year, adjusted to cost per serving.
2. The cost of food for meals for each of the 5 days was calculated as the weighted average of costs on the basis of the number of servings of each item and the number of meals served. In this example, the (weighted) average meal and food cost based on the 5 days of menus was \$0.818 (see "Weekly Means" in Appendix M). This weighted average was estimated from a range of costs (\$0.616 to \$0.959 per meal).
3. The costs then were adjusted by the CPI-FAFH, yielding an average food cost of \$1.07 per meal for 2006 and \$1.16 per meal for 2008 (see numbers in boldface at the bottom of Appendix M).

Notably, the average SFA cost of food for the 2005–2006 school year for a reimbursable meal was \$1.09, \$0.02 higher than the committee's estimate for 2006.

Advantages and Limitations of the Proposed Overall Approach

The advantage of the proposed overall approach to estimating cost implications is that it is feasible and allows considerable flexibility in making adjustments to the proposed changes in Meal Requirements as reflected in the menus. However, some limitations should be noted. Price changes over the period are not uniform across all foods. Moreover, new foods and packaging change costs, as do changes in school procurement procedures. These factors will be considered in a qualitative way, and if it is deemed to be necessary, additional adjustments in prices will be made. Such adjustment will be based on the recent experience of school districts in purchasing and implementing practices that are consistent with the proposed revisions of the Nutrition Standards and the Menu Requirements.

Other Considerations

Data on labor, administrative, and other costs will be included on the basis of the 2005–2006 school year estimates from the USDA cost study (USDA, 2008e), as well as relevant information obtained from school districts. Data on variations across SFAs by size and other factors from this recent USDA study will also allow the generation of a range of cost estimates.

The effects of changes in labor and administrative costs will be considered in a qualitative manner, on the basis of the experience of the SFAs and schools that have implemented changes that are consistent with specific recommended changes to the Meal Requirements. In the same way, Phase II will consider changes in indirect costs for labor, equipment, and other items that may not be reported.

The adjustments and changes that the committee tests with this model may have significant cost implications. Further adjustments in the foods included in the base menu may be required to temper projected increases in the cost of food. Such increases may result from decreases in the availability and use of donated commodities and from specific recommended changes to the Nutrition Standards and Meal Requirements. School districts have some experience with implementing changes in school meals and in responding to unexpected market events (product recalls, for example).

Changes in student participation do not directly affect the cost estimates. However, for any proposed change, the committee will consider the potential effect of the change on student participation in the school meal program. That is, a change in the meal offered may induce more (or fewer) students to participate in the school meal program. Another possible effect might be the participation of more (or fewer) students who pay the full price of the meal. Expectations of changes in participation and implications for costs will be based on the experiences of SFAs and schools that have implemented changes that are consistent with the proposed changes.

ESTIMATION OF MARKET EFFECTS

The Phase II report will also include an analysis of the economic impacts of the recommended revisions to the Nutrient Standards and the Meal Requirements on SFAs and commodity markets. The impact of each of the proposed changes will be included and assessed on the basis of the available information.

A USDA study of food costs (USDA, 1998b) that developed a summary of the dollar value of food acquisitions by public unified school districts that participate in the NSLP will provide a starting point. The USDA study provided estimated school expenditures (dollar values) for all foods, purchased foods, processed foods containing donated commodities, and donated commodities for the 1996–1997 school year, as well as the distribution of the costs (dollar values) of different food groups (i.e., the percentage of the total cost spent on grain products, bakery products, etc.). To view the complete list of dollar values, see Table V-II in the School Food Purchase Study (USDA, 1998b). Adjustment for changes in market prices and aggregate school purchase patterns will provide the basis for the development of the analysis of commodity markets.

Proposed changes to the Nutrition Standards and the Meal Requirements will likely have an effect on the foods that are made available through the meals programs. Estimated economic effects on commodity markets will consider the impacts on markets under assumptions of full substitution and full supplementation and the expected levels of substitution and supplementation. Estimates of the expected levels of substitution and supplementation will be based on information available from school districts that have experimented with changes and from the SNDA-III data on foods consumed as school meals (outside of the school meals program) and at home.

Any changes to the Nutrition Standards and the Meal Requirements for the school meal programs will occur in a period of rapidly changing prices. The ability of SFAs to adjust meals and meet relevant standards in such an environment of changing costs is likely to depend on a number of factors, including the school's state and local fiscal environment, the student population and demographics, and local food preferences. In addition, the 2008 Farm Bill proposes significant changes in the commodities available to schools, particularly fruits, vegetables, and whole grains. Under this bill, schools are encouraged to purchase locally grown and locally raised agricultural products, offered grants to provide fruits and vegetables distributed through the Fresh Fruit and Vegetable Program, and provided whole grains and whole grain products for use in the school lunch and breakfast programs (*Food, Conservation, and Energy Act of 2008*, P.L. 110-246 (June 18, 2008): § 4304). The committee will consider implications of relevant legislation. Projection of the expected economic impact in such an environment is difficult. The approach considered will make explicit the assumptions used to anticipate the specific economic impacts of proposed changes in the Nutrition Standards and the Meal Requirements.

SUMMARY

During Phase II, the committee will conduct many analyses in the process of developing its recommendations for the Nutrition Standards and Meal Requirements of the school meal programs. Sensitivity analysis will cover food and nutrient intakes according to the 2005 *Dietary Guidelines for Americans* and the DRIs, the costs and administrative impacts of program operations, acceptance by students, and student participation rates on the basis of the available data and evidence. Using a representative set of current school menus, the committee will examine the cost implications of offering that menu set versus a set of menus planned by using proposed revisions to the Nutrition Standards and the Meal Requirements. The committee anticipates that it will use an iterative process in conjunction with its criteria to develop a final set of recommendations for the Nutrition Standards and Meal Requirements of the NSLP and SBP.

7

References

Adams, M. A., R. L. Pelletier, M. M. Zive, and J. F. Sallis. 2005. Salad bars and fruit and vegetable consumption in elementary schools: A plate waste study. *Journal of the American Dietetic Association* 105(11):1789–1792.

Alaimo, K., C. M. Olson, and E. A. Frongillo, Jr. 2001. Low family income and food insufficiency in relation to overweight in U.S. children: Is there a paradox? *Archives of Pediatrics and Adolescent Medicine* 155(10):1161–1167.

Baker, J. L., L. W. Olsen, and T. I. A. Sørensen. 2007. Childhood body-mass index and the risk of coronary heart disease in adulthood. *New England Journal of Medicine* 357(23):2329–2337.

Bandini, L. G., H. Cyr, A. Must, and W. H. Dietz. 1997. Validity of reported energy intake in preadolescent girls. *American Journal of Clinical Nutrition* 65(4 Supp.):1138S–1141S.

Basch, C. E., S. Shea, R. Arliss, I. R. Contento, J. Rips, B. Gutin, M. Irigoyen, and P. Zybert. 1990. Validation of mothers' reports of dietary intake by four to seven year-old children. *American Journal of Public Health* 80(11):1314–1317.

Baxter, S. D., W. O. Thompson, M. S. Litaker, F. H. A. Frye, and C. H. Guinn. 2002. Low accuracy and low consistency of fourth-graders' school breakfast and school lunch recalls. *Journal of the American Dietetic Association* 102(3):386–395.

Baxter, S. D., J. A. Royer, J. W. Hardin, C. H. Guinn, and A. F. Smith. 2007. Fourth-grade children are less accurate in reporting school breakfast than school lunch during 24-hour dietary recalls. *Journal of Nutrition Education and Behavior* 39(3):126–133.

Beaton, G. H. 1994. Approaches to analysis of dietary data: Relationship between planned analyses and choice of methodology. *American Journal of Clinical Nutrition* 59(1 Suppl.):253S–261S.

Bhattacharya, J., J. Currie, and S. Haider. 2004. Poverty, food insecurity, and nutritional outcomes in children and adults. *Journal of Health Economics* 23(4):839–862.

Braam, L. A. J. L. M., M. C. Ocke, H. B. Bueno-De-Mesquita, and J. C. Seidell. 1998. Determinants of obesity-related underreporting of energy intake. *American Journal of Epidemiology* 147(11):1081–1086.

Briefel, R. R., C. T. Sempos, M. A. McDowell, S. Chien, and K. Alaimo. 1997. Dietary methods research in the third National Health and Nutrition Examination Survey: Underreporting of energy intake. *American Journal of Clinical Nutrition* 65(4 Suppl.):1203S–1209S.

Britten, P., K. Marcoe, S. Yamini, and C. Davis. 2006. Development of food intake patterns for the MyPyramid food guidance system. *Journal of Nutrition Education and Behavior* 38(6 Suppl.):S78–S92.

Burghardt, J. A., B. L. Devaney, and A. R. Gordon. 1995. The school nutrition dietary assessment study: Summary and discussion. *American Journal of Clinical Nutrition* 61(1 Suppl.):252S–257S.

Carriquiry, A. L. 1999. Assessing the prevalence of nutrient inadequacy. *Public Health Nutrition* 2(1):23–33.

Casey, P. H., P. M. Simpson, J. M. Gossett, M. L. Bogle, C. M. Champagne, C. Connell, D. Harsha, B. McCabe-Sellers, J. M. Robbins, J. E. Stuff, and J. Weber. 2006. The association of child and household food insecurity with childhood overweight status. *Pediatrics* 118(5):e1406–e1413.

CDC (Centers for Disease Control and Prevention). 2002. Iron Deficiency—United States, 1999–2000. *Morbidity and Mortality Weekly Report* 51(40):897–899. http://www.cdc.gov/mmwr/preview/mmwrhtml/mm5140a1.htm (accessed October 22, 2008).

CDC. 2003. Physical activity levels among children aged 9–13 years—United States, 2002. *Morbidity and Mortality Weekly Report* 52(33):785–788.

CDC. 2004. Spina bifida and anencephaly before and after folic acid mandate—United States, 1995–1996 and 1999–2000. *Morbidity and Mortality Weekly Report* 53(17):362–365. http://www.cdc.gov/mmwr/preview/mmwrhtml/mm5317a3.htm (accessed October 22, 2008).

CDC. 2008a. *Overweight Prevalence*. http://www.cdc.gov/nccdphp/dnpa/obesity/childhood/prevalence.htm (accessed August 5, 2008).

CDC. 2008b. *School Health Profiles: Characteristics of Health Programs Among Secondary Schools 2006*. Atlanta, GA: CDC. http://www.cdc.gov/healthyyouth/profiles/ (accessed September 2, 2008).

CDC. 2008c. *National Report on Biochemical Indicators of Diet and Nutrition in the U.S. Population: 1999–2002*. NCEH Pub. No. 08-2982c. Atlanta, GA: CDC. http://www.cdc.gov/nutritionreport/download.html (accessed October 27, 2008).

CFPA (California Food Policy Advocates). 2008. *The Federal Child Nutrition Commodity Program: A Report on Nutritional Quality*. Oakland, CA: CFPA. http://www.cfpa.net/School_Food/commodities_full.pdf (accessed September 29, 2008).

Cleveland, L. E., D. A. Cook, S. M. Krebs-Smith, and J. Friday. 1997. Method for assessing food intakes in terms of servings based on food guidance. *American Journal of Clinical Nutrition* 65(Suppl.):1254S–1263S.

Cullen, K. W., K. Watson, and I. Zakeri. 2008. Improvements in middle school student dietary intake after implementation of the Texas Public School Nutrition Policy. *American Journal of Public Health* 98(1):111–117.

De Ferranti, S. D., K. Gauvreau, D. S. Ludwig, J. W. Newburger, and N. Rifai. 2006. Inflammation and changes in metabolic syndrome abnormalities in US adolescents: Findings from the 1988–1994 and 1999–2000 National Health and Nutrition Examination Surveys. *Clinical Chemistry* 52(7):1325–1330.

Devaney, B., P. Ziegler, S. Pac, V. Karwe, and S. I. Barr. 2004. Nutrient intakes of infants and toddlers. *Journal of the American Dietetic Association* 104(Suppl. 1):S14–S21.

Ebbeling, C. B., and D. S. Ludwig. 2008. Tracking pediatric obesity: An index of uncertainty? *Journal of the American Medical Association* 299(20):2442–2443.

Gleason, P. M., and C. W. Suitor. 2003. Eating at school: How the National School Lunch Program affects children's diets. *American Journal of Agricultural Economics* 85(4):1047–1061.

Gordon, A. R., B. L. Devaney, and J. A. Burghardt. 1995. Dietary effects of the National School Lunch Program and the School Breakfast Program. *American Journal of Clinical Nutrition* 61(1 Suppl.):221S–231S.

Goulding, A., R. Cannan, S. M. Williams, E. J. Gold, R. W. Taylor, and N. J. Lewis-Barned. 1998. Bone mineral density in girls with forearm fractures. *Journal of Bone and Mineral Research* 13(1):143–148.

Goulding, A., I. E. Jones, R. W. Taylor, S. M. Williams, and P. J. Manning. 2001. Bone mineral density and body composition in boys with distal forearm fractures: A dual-energy x-ray absorptiometry study. *Journal of Pediatrics* 139(4):509–515.

Greer, F. R., N. F. Krebs, R. D. Baker, Jr., J. J. S. Bhatia, M. B. Heyman, F. Lifshitz, D. Blum-Kemelor, M. P. Boland, W. Dietz, V. S. Hubbard, S. J. Walker, and P. T. Kanda. 2006. Optimizing bone health and calcium intakes of infants, children, and adolescents. *Pediatrics* 117(2):578–585.

Guinn, C. H., S. D. Baxter, J. W. Hardin, J. A. Royer, and A. F. Smith. 2008. Intrusions in children's dietary recalls: The roles of BMI, sex, race, interview protocol, and social desirability. *Obesity* 16(9):2169–2174.

Gundersen, C., B. J. Lohman, J. C. Eisenmann, S. Garasky, and S. D. Stewart. 2008. Child-specific food insecurity and overweight are not associated in a sample of 10- to 15-year-old low-income youth. *Journal of Nutrition* 138(2):371–378.

HHS/USDA (U.S. Department of Health and Human Services/U.S. Department of Agriculture). 1980. *Nutrition and Your Health: Dietary Guidelines for Americans*. Home and Garden Bulletin No. 232. Washington, DC: U.S. Government Printing Office. http://www.cnpp.usda.gov/Publications/DietaryGuidelines/1980/DG1980pub.pdf (accessed July 23, 2008).

HHS/USDA. 1995. *Nutrition and Your Health: Dietary Guidelines for Americans*, 4th ed. Washington, DC: U.S. Government Printing Office. http://www.cnpp.usda.gov/dgaspreviousguidelines1995guidelines.htm (accessed September 2, 2008).

HHS/USDA. 2004. *Report of the Dietary Guidelines Advisory Committee on the Dietary Guidelines for Americans, 2005*. Washington, DC: U.S. Government Printing Office. http://www.health.gov/dietaryguidelines/dga2005/report/ (accessed September 12, 2008).

HHS/USDA. 2005. *Dietary Guidelines for Americans*, 6th ed. Washington, DC: U.S. Government Printing Office. http://www.health.gov/DietaryGuidelines/dga2005/document (accessed July 23, 2008).

IOM (Institute of Medicine). 1997. *Dietary Reference Intakes for Calcium, Phosphorus, Magnesium, Vitamin D, and Fluoride*. Washington, DC: National Academy Press.

IOM. 1998. *Dietary Reference Intakes for Thiamin, Riboflavin, Niacin, Vitamin* B_6, *Folate, Vitamin* B_{12}, *Pantothenic Acid, Biotin, and Choline*. Washington, DC: National Academy Press.

IOM. 2000a. *Dietary Reference Intakes for Vitamin C, Vitamin E, Selenium, and Carotenoids*. Washington, DC: National Academy Press.

IOM. 2000b. *Dietary Reference Intakes: Applications in Dietary Assessment*. Washington, DC: National Academy Press.

IOM. 2001. *Dietary Reference Intakes for Vitamin A, Vitamin K, Arsenic, Boron, Chromium, Copper, Iodine, Iron, Manganese, Molybdenum, Nickel, Silicon, Vanadium, and Zinc*. Washington, DC: National Academy Press.

IOM. 2002/2005. *Dietary Reference Intakes for Energy, Carbohydrate, Fiber, Fat, Fatty Acids, Cholesterol, Protein, and Amino Acids (Macronutrients)*. Washington, DC: The National Academies Press.

IOM. 2003. *Dietary Reference Intakes: Applications in Dietary Planning*. Washington, DC: The National Academies Press.

IOM. 2005. *Dietary Reference Intakes for Water, Potassium, Sodium, Chloride, and Sulfate*. Washington, DC: The National Academies Press.

IOM. 2006a. *Food Insecurity and Hunger in the United States: An Assessment of the Measure*. Washington, DC: The National Academies Press.

IOM. 2006b. *Dietary Reference Intakes: The Essential Guide to Nutrient Requirements*. Washington, DC: The National Academies Press.

IOM. 2007. *Nutrition Standards for Foods in Schools: Leading the Way Toward Healthier Youth*. Washington, DC: The National Academies Press.

ISU (Iowa State University). 1997. *Software for Intake Distribution Estimation (PC-SIDE)*, Version 1.02. Ames: ISU.

Jago, R., J. S. Harrell, R. G. McMurray, S. Edelstein, L. El Ghormli, and S. Bassin. 2006. Prevalence of abnormal lipid and blood pressure values among an ethnically diverse population of eighth-grade adolescents and screening implications. *Pediatrics* 117(6):2065–2073.

Johnson, R. K., B. A. Yon, and J. H. Hankin. 2008. Dietary assessment and validation. In *Research: Successful Approaches*, 3rd ed., edited by E. R. Monsen and L. Van Horn. Chicago, IL: American Dietetic Association.

Kennedy, E., and C. Davis. 1998. U.S. Department of Agriculture School Breakfast Program. *American Journal of Clinical Nutrition* 67(4):798S–803S.

Little, P., J. Barnett, B. Margetts, A. L. Kinmonth, J. Gabbay, R. Thompson, D. Warm, H. Warwick, and S. Wooton. 1999. The validity of dietary assessment in general practice. *Journal of Epidemiology and Community Health* 53(3):165–172.

Livingstone, M. B. E., A. M. Prentice, W. A. Coward, J. J. Strain, A. E. Black, P. S. W. Davies, C. M. Stewart, P. G. McKenna, and R. G. Whitehead. 1992. Validation of estimates of energy intake by weighed dietary record and diet history in children and adolescents. *American Journal of Clinical Nutrition* 56(1):29–35.

Lytle, L. A., M. Z. Nichaman, E. Obarzanek, E. Glovsky, D. Montgomery, T. Nicklas, M. Zive, and H. Feldman. 1993. Validation of 24-hour recalls assisted by food records in third-grade children. *Journal of the American Dietetic Association* 93(12):1431–1436.

Marcoe, K., W. Juan, S. Yamini, A. Carlson, and P. Britten. 2006. Development of food group composites and nutrient profiles for the MyPyramid food guidance system. *Journal of Nutrition Education and Behavior* 38(6 Suppl.):S93–S107.

Marples, C. A., and D. M. Spillman. 1995. Factors affecting students' participation in the Cincinnati public schools lunch program. *Adolescence* 30(119):745–754.

Martin, J. 2008a. Overview of the federal child nutrition legislation. In *Managing Child Nutrition Programs: Leadership for Excellence*, 2nd ed., edited by J. Martin and C. B. Oakley. Boston, MA: Jones and Bartlett Publishers. Pp. 145–202.

Martin, J. 2008b. History of child nutrition programs. In *Managing Child Nutrition Programs: Leadership for Excellence*, 2nd ed., edited by J. Martin and C. B. Oakley. Boston, MA: Jones and Bartlett Publishers. Pp. 47–143.

Martin, K. S., and A. M. Ferris. 2007. Food insecurity and gender are risk factors for obesity. *Journal of Nutrition Education and Behavior* 39(1):31–36.

Messiah, S. E., K. L. Arheart, B. Luke, S. E. Lipshultz, and T. L. Miller. 2008. Relationship between body mass index and metabolic syndrome risk factors among U.S. 8- to 14-year-olds, 1999 to 2002. *Journal of Pediatrics* 153(2):215–221.

Moshfegh, A. J., D. G. Rhodes, D. J. Baer, T. Murayi, J. C. Clemens, W. V. Rumpler, D. R. Paul, R. S. Sebastian, K. J. Kuczynski, L. A. Ingwersen, R. C. Staples, and L. E. Cleveland. 2008. The US Department of Agriculture Automated Multiple-Pass Method reduces bias in the collection of energy intakes. *American Journal of Clinical Nutrition* 88(2):324–332.

NCH (National Coalition for the Homeless). 2008. *Homeless Families with Children: NCH Fact Sheet #12*. http://www.nationalhomeless.org/publications/facts/families.html (accessed October 29, 2008).

NRC (National Research Council). 1986. *Nutrient Adequacy: Assessment Using Food Consumption Surveys*. Washington, DC: National Academy Press.

NRC. 1989. *Recommended Dietary Allowances*, 10th ed. Washington, DC: National Academy Press.

Nusser, S. M., A. L. Carriquiry, K. W. Dodd, and W. A. Fuller. 1996. A semiparametric transformation approach to estimating usual daily intake distributions. *Journal of the American Statistical Association* 91(436):1440–1449.

Ogden, C. L., M. D. Carroll, and K. M. Flegal. 2008. High body mass index for age among U.S. children and adolescents, 2003–2006. *Journal of the American Medical Association* 299(20):2401–2405.

Pryer, J. A., M. Vrijheid, R. Nichols, M. Kiggins, and P. Elliott. 1997. Who are the "low energy reporters" in the Dietary and Nutritional Survey of British Adults? *International Journal of Epidemiology* 26(1):146–154.

SNA (School Nutrition Association). 2007. *School Nutrition Operations Report: The State of School Nutrition 2007*. Alexandria, VA: SNA.

SNA/SNF (School Nutrition Association/School Nutrition Foundation). 2007. *From Cupcakes to Carrots: Local Wellness Policies One Year Later*. Alexandria, VA: SNA.

Stallone, D. D., E. J. Brunner, S. A. Bingham, and M. G. Marmot. 1997. Dietary assessment in Whitehall II: The influence of reporting bias on apparent socioeconomic variation in nutrient intakes. *European Journal of Clinical Nutrition* 51(12):815–825.

U.S. Bureau of Labor Statistics. 2008. *Consumer Price Index Database: All Urban Consumers*. http://www.bls.gov/cpi/data.htm (accessed September 22, 2008).

U.S. Census Bureau. 2006. Table C3. Living Arrangements of Children Under 18 Years and Marital Status of Parents, by Age, Gender, Race, and Hispanic Origin of the Child for All Children: 2006. In *America's Families and Living Arrangements: 2006*. http://www.census.gov/population/www/socdemo/hh-fam/cps2006.html (accessed August 28, 2008).

U.S. Department of Education. 2000a. *The Release of the Condition of Education: 2000*. http://nces.ed.gov/whatsnew/commissioner/remarks2000/6_01_2000.asp (accessed October 24, 2008).

U.S. Department of Education. 2000b. *In the Middle: Characteristics of Public Schools with a Focus on Middle Schools.* Report NCES 2000-312. Washington, DC: National Center for Education Statistics. http://nces.ed.gov/pubSearch/pubsinfo.asp?pubid=2000312 (accessed September 12, 2008).

U.S. Department of Education. 2004. *Education for Homeless Children and Youth Program: Title VII-B of the McKinney-Vento Homeless Assistance Act, as amended by the No Child Left Behind Act of 2001 Non-Regulatory Guidance.* Washington, DC: U.S. Department of Educations. http://www.ed.gov/programs/homeless/guidance.pdf (accessed October 1, 2008).

U.S. Department of Education. 2007. *Public Elementary and Secondary School Student Enrollment, High School Completions, and Staff from the Common Core of Data: School Year 2005-06. First Look.* Report NCES 2007-352. Washington, DC: National Center for Education Statistics. http://nces.ed.gov/pubsearch/pubsinfo.asp?pubid=2007352 (accessed August 22, 2008).

U.S. Department of Education. 2008a. *Digest of Education Statistics 2007.* Report NCES 2008-022. Washington, DC: National Center for Education Statistics. http://nces.ed.gov/pubs 2008/2008022.pdf (accessed August 22, 2008).

U.S. Department of Education. 2008b. *Characteristics of the 100 Largest Public Elementary and Secondary School Districts in the United States: 2005–06.* Report NCES 2008-339. Washington, DC: National Center for Education Statistics. http://nces.ed.gov/pubs2008/ 2008339.pdf (accessed August 22, 2008).

USDA (U.S. Department of Agriculture). 1976. Part 210—National School Lunch Program. *Federal Register* 41(114):23695–23696.

USDA. 1993. *The School Nutrition Dietary Assessment Study: School Food Service, Meals Offered, and Dietary Intakes.* Alexandria, VA: USDA, Food and Nutrition Service. http://www.fns.usda.gov/OANE/MENU/Published/CNP/cnp-archive.htm (accessed August 4, 2008).

USDA. 1994a. National School Lunch Program and School Breakfast Program: Nutrition objectives for school meals; proposed rule. *Federal Register* 59(111):30217–30251.

USDA. 1994b. *School Lunch and Breakfast Cost Study: Executive Summary.* http://www.fns. usda.gov/OANE/MENU/Published/CNP/FILES/LunchandBreakfastCost.htm (accessed August 4, 2008).

USDA. 1995. National School Lunch Program and School Breakfast Program: School meals initiative for healthy children: Final Rule. *Federal Register* 60(113):31188–31222.

USDA. 1997. *Evaluation of the Nutrient Standard Menu Planning Demonstration: Findings from the Formative Evaluation.* Alexandria, VA: USDA, Food and Nutrition Service. http://www.fns.usda.gov/oane/menu/Published/CNP/FILES/formev2.pdf (accessed August 6, 2008).

USDA. 1998a. *Evaluation of the Nutrient Standard Menu Planning Demonstration: Summary of Findings.* Alexandria, VA: USDA, Food and Nutrition Service. http://www.fns.usda.gov/ oane/menu/Published/CNP/FILES/nsmpdem.pdf (accessed August 6, 2008).

USDA. 1998b. *School Food Purchase Study: Final Report.* Alexandria, VA: USDA, Food and Nutrition Service. http://www.fns.usda.gov/OANE/MENU/Published/CNP/cnp-archive. htm (accessed August 4, 2008).

USDA. 1998c. *Eating Breakfast: Effects of the School Breakfast Program.* Alexandria, VA: USDA, Food and Nutrition Service. Http://www.fns.usda.gov/OANE/MENU/Published/CNP/FILES/BR-REP.PDF (accessed August 4, 2008).

USDA. 1999. *The Story of Team Nutrition: Executive Summary of the Pilot Study.* Alexandria, VA: USDA, Food and Nutrition Service. http://www.fns.usda.gov/oane/menu/Published/CNP/FILES/tn2execsum.pdf (accessed August 5, 2008).

USDA. 2000a. *The School Meals Initiative Implementation Study—First Year Report.* Alexandria, VA: USDA, Food and Nutrition Service. http://www.fns.usda.gov/oane/menu/Published/CNP/FILES/SMIYear1.pdf (accessed August 5, 2008).

USDA. 2000b. *Meal Planning in the National School Lunch Program.* Alexandria, VA: USDA, Food and Nutrition Service. http://www.fns.usda.gov/cnd/menu/menu.planning.NSLP.htm (accessed August 26, 2008).

USDA. 2001a. *School Nutrition Dietary Assessment Study—II Final Report.* Alexandria, VA: USDA, Food and Nutrition Service. http://www.fns.usda.gov/OANE/MENU/Published/CNP/FILES/sndaII.pdf (accessed August 4, 2008).

USDA. 2001b. *The School Meals Initiative Implementation Study—Second Year Report.* Alexandria, VA: USDA, Food and Nutrition Service. http://www.fns.usda.gov/oane/menu/Published/CNP/FILES/smiy2.pdf (accessed August 5, 2008).

USDA. 2001c. National School Lunch Program and School Breakfast Program: Alternatives to standard application and meal counting procedures. *Federal Register* 66(183):48323–48334.

USDA. 2002a. *The School Meals Initiative Implementation Study—Third Year Report.* Alexandria, VA: USDA, Food and Nutrition Service. http://www.fns.usda.gov/oane/menu/Published/CNP/FILES/smiyear3.pdf (accessed August 4, 2008).

USDA. 2002b. *School Lunch Salad Bars.* Alexandria, VA: USDA, Food and Nutrition Service. http://www.fns.usda.gov/OANE/MENU/Published/CNP/FILES/saladbar.pdf (accessed August 8, 2008).

USDA. 2002c. *Provision 2 Guidance: National School Lunch and School Breakfast Programs.* Alexandria, VA: USDA, Food and Nutrition Service. http://www.fns.usda.gov/cnd/Governance/prov-1-2-3/Prov2Guidance.pdf (accessed October 21, 2008).

USDA. 2004. *Evaluation of the School Breakfast Program Pilot Project: Final Report.* Alexandria, VA: USDA, Food and Nutrition Service. http://www.fns.usda.gov/OANE/MENU/Published/CNP/FILES/SBPPFinal.pdf (accessed August 4, 2008).

USDA. 2005. *MyPyramid Food Intake Patterns.* http://www.mypyramid.gov/professional/pdf_food_intake.html (accessed August 7, 2008).

USDA. 2006a. *USDA-approved Software Requirements Regarding Vitamin A.* http://www.fns.usda.gov/CND/Governance/Policy-Memos/2006/SP_24-2006.pdf (accessed October 21, 2008).

USDA. 2006b. *MyPyramid Equivalents Database for USDA Survey Food Codes, 1994–2002,* Version 1.0. http://www.ars.usda.gov/Services/docs.htm?docid=8503 (accessed August 8, 2008).

USDA. 2007a. *School Nutrition Dietary Assessment Study—III.* Alexandria, VA: USDA, Food and Nutrition Service. http://www.fns.usda.gov/oane/MENU/Published/recentreleases.htm (accessed August 4, 2008).

USDA. 2007b. *The Road to SMI Success: A Guide for Food Service Directors*. Alexandria, VA: USDA, Food and Nutrition Service. http://www.fns.usda.gov/tn/Resources/roadtosuccess.html (accessed August 22, 2008).

USDA. 2007c. *Food Distribution Programs: History and Background*. http://www.fns.usda.gov/fdd/aboutfd/history.htm (accessed October 2, 2008).

USDA. 2007d. *USDA Commodities in the National School Lunch Program*. Alexandria, VA: USDA, Food and Nutrition Service. http://www.fns.usda.gov/fdd/foods/healthy/WhitePaper.pdf (accessed October 31, 2008).

USDA. 2008a. *The National School Lunch Program Background and Development*. http://www.fns.usda.gov/cnd/Lunch/AboutLunch/ProgramHistory_5.htm (accessed August 15, 2008).

USDA. 2008b. *The National School Lunch Program: Background, Trends, and Issues*. http://www.ers.usda.gov/Publications/ERR61/ (accessed August 4, 2008).

USDA. 2008c. *National School Lunch Program: Participation and Lunches Served*. http://www.fns.usda.gov/pd/slsummar.htm (accessed August 5, 2008).

USDA. 2008d. *School Breakfast Program Participation and Meals Served*. http://www.fns.usda.gov/pd/sbsummar.htm (accessed August 5, 2008).

USDA. 2008e. *School Lunch and Breakfast Cost Study—II, Final Report*. Alexandria, VA: USDA, Food and Nutrition Service. http://www.fns.usda.gov/OANE/MENU/Published/CNP/FILES/MealCostStudy.pdf (accessed August 4, 2008).

USDA. 2008f. *Menu Planning in the School Breakfast Program*. Alexandria, VA: USDA, Food and Nutrition Service. http://www.fns.usda.gov/cnd/Breakfast/Menu/sbp-menu-planning.htm (accessed August 26, 2008).

USDA. 2008g. *Federal Cost of School Food Programs*. http://www.fns.usda.gov/pd/cncosts.htm (accessed October 7, 2008).

USDA. 2008h. National School Lunch, Special Milk, and School Breakfast Programs, National average payments/maximum reimbursement rates. *Federal Register* 73(130):38392–38395.

USDA. 2008i. *Schools/Child Nutrition Commodity Programs*. Alexandria, VA: USDA, Food and Nutrition Service. http://www.fns.usda.gov/fdd/programs/schcnp/pfs-schcnp.pdf (accessed September 29, 2008).

USDA. 2008j. *About Commodity Processing*. http://www.fns.usda.gov/fdd/processing/about_processing.htm (accessed August 5, 2008).

USDA. 2008k. *Food Distribution Programs: Department of Defense Fresh Fruit and Vegetable Program*. http://www.fns.usda.gov/fdd/programs/dod/DoD_FreshFruitandVegetableProgram.pdf (accessed September 29, 2008).

USDA. 2008l. *Diet Quality of American School-Age Children by School Lunch Participation Status: Data from the National Health and Nutrition Examination Survey, 1999–2004*. Alexandria, VA: USDA, Food and Nutrition Service. http://www.fns.usda.gov/OANE/menu/published/CNP/FILES/NHANES-NSLP.pdf (accessed August 20, 2008).

USDA. 2008m. *Child Nutrition Labeling*. http://www.fns.usda.gov/cnd/cnlabeling/default.htm (accessed August 6, 2008).

USDA. 2008n. *Inside the Pyramid*. http://www.mypyramid.gov/pyramid/index.html (accessed October 24, 2008).

USDA. 2008o. *Diet Quality of Americans by Food Stamp Participation Status: Data from the National Health and Nutrition Examination Survey, 1999–2004*. Alexandria, VA: Food and Nutrition Service, USDA. http://www.fns.usda.gov/OANE/menu/published/FSP/FILES/Participation/NHANES-FSP.pdf (accessed September 10, 2008).

USDA/ARS (U.S. Department of Agriculture/Agricultural Research Service). 2004. *USDA Food and Nutrient Database for Dietary Studies*, Version 1.0. http://www.ars.usda.gov/Services/docs.htm?docid=12082 (accessed September 10, 2008).

USDA/ARS. 2005. *What We Eat in America, NHANES 2001–2002: Usual Nutrient Intakes from Food Compared to Dietary Reference Intakes*. Washington, DC: USDA/ARS. http://www.ars.usda.gov/Services/docs.htm?docid=15045 (accessed September 29, 2008).

USDA/ARS. 2008. *USDA National Nutrient Database for Standard Reference*, Release 20. http://www.ars.usda.gov/research/publications/publications.htm?seq_no_115=214178 (accessed September 10, 2008).

USDA/ERS (U.S. Department of Agriculture/Economic Research Service). 2004. *Effects of Food Assistance and Nutrition Programs on Nutrition and Health*, Vol. 4. *Executive Summary of the Literature Review*. Food Assistance and Nutrition Research Report Number 19-4. Washington, DC: USDA, ERS. http://www.ers.usda.gov/Publications/FANRR19-4/ (accessed August 18, 2008).

USDA/ERS. 2006. *Household Food Security in the United States, 2005*. Economic Research Report Number 29. Washington, DC: USDA, ERS. http://www.ers.usda.gov/Publications/ERR29/ (accessed August 20, 2008).

USDA/ERS. 2007a. *Food Security in the United States: Hunger and Food Security*. http://www.ers.usda.gov/briefing/foodsecurity/labels.htm (accessed October 30, 2008).

USDA/ERS. 2007b. *Review of Dietary Reference Intakes for Selected Nutrients: Challenges and Implications for Federal Food and Nutrition Policy*. Contractor and Cooperator Report Number 28. Washington, DC: USDA/ERS. http://www.ers.usda.gov/publications/ccr28/ccr28.pdf (accessed September 10, 2008).

USDA/ERS. 2008. *The Food Assistance Landscape: FY 2007 Annual Report*. Washington, DC: USDA, Economic Research Service. http://www.ers.usda.gov/Publications/EIB6-5/ (accessed August 28, 2008).

Ventura, A. K., E. Loken, D. C. Mitchell, H. Smiciklas-Wright, and L. L. Birch. 2006. Understanding reporting bias in the dietary recall data of 11-year-old girls. *Obesity* 14(6):1073–1084.

Wechsler, H., C. E. Basch, P. Zybert, and S. Shea. 1998. Promoting the selection of low-fat milk in elementary school cafeterias in an inner-city Latino community: Evaluation of an intervention. *American Journal of Public Health* 88(3):427–433.

Wellisch, J., S. D. Hanes, L. A. Jordon, K. M. Mauer, and J. A. Vermeersch. 1983. *The National Evaluation of School Nutrition Programs*, Vol. 1 and 2. Santa Monica, CA: Systems Development Corporation.

Wojcicki, J. M., and M. B. Heyman. 2006. Healthier choices and increased participation in a middle school lunch program: Effects of nutrition policy changes in San Francisco. *American Journal of Public Health* 96(9):1542–1547.

Wyshak, G., and R. E. Frisch. 1994. Carbonated beverages, dietary calcium, the dietary calcium/phosphorus ratio, and bone fractures in girls and boys. *Journal of Adolescent Health* 15(3):210–215.

Yetley, E. A. 2008. Assessing the vitamin D status of the U.S. population. *American Journal of Clinical Nutrition* 88(2):558S–564S.

Appendix A

Acronyms, Abbreviations, and Glossary

ACRONYMS AND ABBREVIATIONS

AI	Adequate Intake
AMDR	Acceptable Macronutrient Distribution Range
AMS	Agricultural Marketing Service, U.S. Department of Agriculture
ARS	Agricultural Research Service, U.S. Department of Agriculture
BMI	body mass index
CDC	Centers for Disease Control and Prevention
CFR	*Code of Federal Regulations*
CN	Child nutrition
CNP	Child Nutrition Programs
CPI	Consumer Price Index
DASH	Dietary Approaches to Stop Hypertension
DFE	dietary folate equivalent
DGA	Dietary Guidelines for Americans
DRI	Dietary Reference Intakes
EAR	Estimated Average Requirement
EER	Estimated Energy Requirement
FAFH	food away from home
FBMP	food-based menu planning
FNDDS	Food and Nutrient Database for Dietary Studies
FNS	Food and Nutrition Service, U.S. Department of Agriculture
FY	fiscal year
g	gram
G/B	grain/bread
HHS	U.S. Department of Health and Human Services
IOM	Institute of Medicine, The National Academies
IU	international unit
K	kindergarten
kcal	kilocalorie/calorie
mg	milligram

M/MA	meat/meat alternate
NBMP	nutrient-based menu planning
NCHS	National Center for Health Statistics, Centers for Disease Control and Prevention
NHANES	National Health and Nutrition Examination Survey
NSLA	National School Lunch Act
NSLP	National School Lunch Program
OVS	offer versus serve
oz	ounce
P.L.	Public Law
PPS	probability proportional to size
RA/RAE	retinol activity/retinol activity equivalent
RDA	Recommended Dietary Allowance
RE	retinol equivalent
REA	Recommended Energy Allowance
SBP	School Breakfast Program
SFA	school food authority
SMI	School Meals Initiative
SNDA	School Nutrition and Dietary Assessment Study
TMI	target median intake
tsp	teaspoon
μg	microgram
UL	Tolerable Upper Intake Level
USDA	U.S. Department of Agriculture
V/F	vegetable/fruit
WIC	Special Supplemental Nutrition Program for Women, Infants, and Children

GLOSSARY

Acceptable Macronutrient Distribution Ranges The range of intakes of an energy source that is associated with a reduced risk of chronic disease yet that can provide adequate amounts of essential nutrients.

Adequate Intake A recommended average daily nutrient intake level based on observed or experimentally determined approximations or estimates of nutrient intake by a group or groups of apparently healthy people that are assumed to be adequate.

Alternate Menu Planning Approaches (Any Reasonable Approach) Menu planning approaches that are adopted or developed by state food authorities or state agencies and that differ from the standard approaches. The state agency should be contacted for specific details, as alternate approaches may require prior state agency review and approval.

Assisted Nutrient Standard Menu Planning Approach One of the nutrient-based menu planning approaches that provides schools with menus developed and nutritionally analyzed by other sources. These sources may include the state agency, other state food agencies authorities, consultants, or food service management companies. The supplier of the assisted nutrient standard menus must also develop and provide recipes, food product specifications, and preparation techniques.

Dietary Reference Intakes A family of nutrient reference values.

Enhanced Food-Based Menu Planning Approach One of the two food-based menu planning approaches established by the U.S. Department of Agriculture that uses meal patterns with food items from specific food group components in specific amounts, by age-grade group, to plan meals. It is similar to the traditional food-based menu planning approach, except that it uses different age-grade groups and a different number of servings of vegetables/fruits and grains/breads.

Entrée Under the nutrient-based menu planning approaches, an entrée is a school lunch menu item that is a combination of foods or a single food item offered as the main course, as defined by the menu planner. The entrée is the central focus of the meal and forms the framework around which the rest of the meal is planned.

Estimated Average Requirement The usual daily intake level that is estimated to meet the requirement of half the healthy individuals in a life-stage and gender group.

Estimated Energy Requirement For children, the estimated energy requirement represents the sum of the dietary energy intake predicted to maintain energy balance for the child's age, weight, height, and activity level plus an amount to cover normal growth and development.

Food-Based Menu Planning One of two approaches used to implement the Nutrition Standards. It focuses on types and amounts of foods. Food-based menu planning, as established by the U.S. Department of Agriculture, includes so-called traditional and enhanced approaches.

Food Component One of four food groups that comprise reimbursable meals planned under a food-based menu-planning approach. The four food components are meat/meat alternate, grains/breads, fruits/vegetables, and fluid milk.

Food Item One of the five foods from the four food components required to be offered in school lunches under food-based menu planning approaches or one of the four foods required to be offered in school breakfasts.

Indicator Nutrients See *Nutrition Standards*

Key Nutrients See *Nutrition Standards*

Meal Patterns A term used to refer to food items under the food-based menu planning approach as specified for various age-grade groups.

Meal Requirements The set of standards used to develop menus and meals so as to implement the Nutrition Standards. Meal Requirements may be met through either food-based menu planning approaches or nutrient-based menu planning approaches.

Menu Item Any single food or combination of foods, except condiments, served in a meal under the nutrient-based menu planning approaches (nutrient standard menu planning and assisted nutrient standard menu planning approaches). All menu items or foods offered as part of the reimbursable meal will be counted toward meeting the nutrition standards.

National School Lunch Program The program under which participating schools operate a nonprofit lunch program, in accordance with 7 CFR Part 210.

Nonreimbursable Meals Meals that are served but that cannot be claimed for reimbursement in the National School Lunch Program and the School Breakfast Program, such as adult meals, à la carte meals, and second meals served to students.

Nutrient Analysis The process of developing or monitoring school menus on the basis of an analysis of the nutrients in the menu items and foods offered over a school week to determine if the specific levels of a set of key nutrients and calories are met for the applicable age-grade group.

Nutrient-Based Menu Planning One of two approaches used to implement the Nutrition Standards. It makes use of computer software to plan menus consistent with the Nutrition Standards. As established by the U.S. Department of Agriculture, the approach includes the so-called nutrient standard approach and the assisted approach.

Nutrient Standards See *Nutrition Standards*

Nutrients and Other Dietary Components A term used to refer collectively to any nutrition-related substance that may be encompassed by the Nutrition Standards, including calories, vitamins, minerals, food components such as saturated fat and whole grains, and food categories such as fruits and vegetables.

Nutrients of Concern See *Nutrition Standards*

Nutrition Standards A collective term for the nutrition goals for school meals that currently includes nutrients and other dietary components that are required as well as those that are recommended. For this report, nutrient standards are encompassed by the Nutrition Standards.

Other related terms:

Indicator Nutrients Term used to refer to nutrients in the Nutrition Standards (or in other government provisions and programs) for which there may not be concerns about adequate or excessive intake but that serve as a proxy for foods and dietary patterns likely to include a range of important nutrients. The term was not specifically used by the U.S. Department of Agriculture in the 1995 implementing regulations.

Key Nutrients The required components of the Nutrition Standards for which minimum requirements for school meals have been established by the U.S. Department of Agriculture. These are calories, calories from total fat, calories from saturated fat, protein, calcium, iron, vitamin A, and vitamin C.

Nutrient Standards Quantitative values derived by using special calculations to quantify the amounts of the key nutrients within the Nutrition Standards for age-grade groups on the basis of a 5-day average.

Nutrients of Concern A term that has evolved over time to refer to nutrients for which there are indications that current intakes are too low or too high. It was not specifically used by U.S. Department of Agriculture in the 1995 regulations for school meals.

Offer Versus Serve For lunch, offer versus serve is required in high school but is optional in junior high and elementary schools. Offer versus serve is optional in all grades for breakfast.

For Food-Based Menu Planning Approaches High school students must be offered a complete lunch of at least five food items, but they may select three full portions of the items for the meal to be qualified for reimbursement. For junior high and elementary schools, students can be required to select either three or four food items. Under offer versus serve, a reimbursable breakfast must contain four food items, from which the student must choose at least three full portions.

For Nutrient-Based Menu Planning Approaches Children must be offered the planned lunch that meets the Nutrition Standard and that includes, at a minimum, an entrée, fluid milk as a beverage, and at least one side dish. If the planned lunch contains three menu items, students can decline one menu item (they cannot decline the entrée). If the planned lunch contains more than three menu items, students cannot decline more than two. A reimbursable breakfast must be the planned breakfast that meets the Nutrition Standard and that contains a minimum of three menu items, one of which must be fluid milk, from which children may decline any one item.

Planning Model The explanation and rationale for the approach used to establish the Nutrition Standards.

Recommended Dietary Allowances The average daily dietary nutrient intake level that is sufficient to meet the nutrient requirements of nearly all (97–98 percent) healthy individuals in a particular life-stage and gender group.

Reimbursable Meal A school meal that meets the U.S. Department of Agriculture Meal Requirements and Nutrition Standard, that is served to an eligible student, and that is priced as an entire meal rather than priced on the basis of individual items. Such meals qualify for reimbursement with federal funds.

School Breakfast Program The program under which participating schools operate a nonprofit breakfast program in accordance with 7 CFR Part 220.

School Food Authority The governing body that is responsible for the administration of one or more schools and that has the legal authority to operate the school meal programs therein or that is otherwise approved by the Food and Nutrition Service of the U.S. Department of Agriculture to operate the school meal programs.

School Meals Initiative The School Meals Initiative includes the regulations that define how the *Dietary Guidelines for Americans* and other Nutrition Standards apply to school meals. This initiative includes actions that support state agencies, school food authorities, and communities in improving school meals and encouraging children to improve their overall diets.

Schoolchildren Children in the United States who are school age (4–18 years old).

Side Dish(es) Any menu item (except condiments) that is offered in addition to the entrée and fluid milk under the nutrient-based menu planning approaches for the school lunch or any menu item offered in addition to fluid milk for the school breakfast.

State Agency State agency refers to (1) the state educational agency or (2) any other agency of the state that has been designated by the governor or other appropriate executive or legislative authority of the state and approved by the U.S. Department of Agriculture to administer the program in schools.

Target Median Intake Statistically derived target intake for nutrients used to plan diets for groups.

Tolerable Upper Intake Level The highest daily nutrient intake level that is likely to pose no risk of adverse health effects to almost all individuals in the general population.

Traditional Food-Based Menu Planning Approach One of the two food-based menu planning approaches established by the U.S. Department of Agriculture that use meal patterns with food items from specific food components in quantities appropriate for established age-grade groups.

Usual Nutrient Intake Data based on 24-hour recall and statistically adjusted to better estimate usual intake; for this report, reference to nutrient intake includes energy (calories).

Appendix B

A Selection of Laws and Regulations Governing the National School Lunch Program and School Breakfast Program

Year	Law or Regulation	Outcome
1946	Richard B. Russell National School Lunch Act, P.L. 79-396	Established the National School Lunch Program (NSLP) as a permanent program
1949	Agricultural Act of 1949, Section 416, P.L. 81-439	Granted authority to the Commodity Credit Corporation to donate commodities to various agencies, including the school lunch programs
1966	Child Nutrition Act of 1966, P.L. 89-642	Began the School Breakfast Program (SBP) as a pilot project
1970	National School Lunch and Child Nutrition Act Amendments, P.L. 91-248	Authorized special assistance fund for all schools serving free and reduced-price lunches, established uniform national guidelines to determine eligibility for free and reduced-price meals, and included several other key elements
1973	Definition of "milk," *Federal Register*, 38:21777, August 13, 1973	Allowed schools to serve low-fat or skim milk
1975	Amendments to the National School Lunch Act and the Child Nutrition Act, P.L. 94-105	Amended the Child Nutrition Act to make the SBP permanent; mandated offer versus serve (OVS) to reduce food waste in the NSLP
1976	Implementation Rule, *Federal Register*, 41:23695, June 11, 1976	Dropped butter and fortified margarine as part of the school lunch meal pattern; established OVS in high schools participating in the NSLP
1977	National School Lunch Act and Child Nutrition Amendments P.L. 95-166	Authorized OVS for middle and junior high schools at the discretion of the school food authority

1978	Nutritional Requirements (Interim Rule), Federal Register, 43:37166, August 22, 1978	Required school lunches to meet one-third of the Recommended Dietary Allowances (RDAs) over a week's time
1980	NSLP; Nutritional Requirements (Final Rule), Federal Register, 45:32502, May 16, 1980	Recommended (not required) that schools vary portion sizes for four age groups: 1–2 years, 3–4 years, grades kindergarten–3 (ages 5–8), and grades 4–12 (ages 9 years and older); recommended larger portion sizes for grades 7–12; schools allowed to serve one meal pattern for all children in grades 4–12
1981	Omnibus Reconciliation Act, P.L. 97-35	Created substantial reductions in meal reimbursement rates and commodity assistance; increased the charges to students for reduced-price lunches (from $0.20 to $0.40) and reduced-price breakfasts (from $0.10 to $0.30); expanded OVS to elementary schools and preschools at the discretion of the school food authority
1986	Amendments to the National School Lunch Act and Child Nutrition Act, P.L. 99-591	Extended the OVS option to school breakfasts
1988	Amendment of the National School Lunch Act, P.L. 100-135	Added three cents to the school breakfast rate
1987	Commodity Distribution and Reform Act, P.L. 100-237	Focused on the quality of commodities and authorized the testing of cash in lieu of commodities or commodity letter of credit
1989	1989 Reauthorization Act, P.L. 101-147	Provided start-up money for the initiation of breakfast programs
1994	Healthy Meals for Healthy Americans Act, P.L. 103-448, Sec.106(b)	Required that the NSLP and the SBP meals meet the Dietary Guidelines for Americans as they evolve; requires the use of a variety of meal-planning approaches, including food-based methods
1995	National School Lunch and School Breakfast Programs: School Meal Initiatives for Healthy Children (Final Rule), Federal Register, 60:31188, June 13, 1995	Allowed nutrient-based and food-based menu planning; revised the meal pattern by increasing the quantities of vegetables/fruits and grains and phased out the traditional meal pattern; set nutrition standards based on the Dietary Guidelines for Americans and the 1989 RDAs; established specific minimum standards for key nutrients and calories; established the following age-grade groups: prekindergarten, kindergarten–6, 7–12, optional kindergarten–3

1996	Healthy Meals for Children Act of 1996, P.L.104-149	Authorized the use of the traditional meal pattern and any other reasonable approach
1996	Personal Responsibility and Work Opportunity Reconciliation Act, P.L. 104-193	Required that lunches and breakfasts provide one-third and one-half of RDAs over a week, respectively (required by existing program regulation)
1998	William F. Goodling Child Nutrition Reauthorization Act of 1998, P.L. 105-336	Authorized pilot programs for universal breakfast programs in some elementary schools and extended pilot programs for universal lunch programs and the commodity programs
2000	National School Lunch Program and School Breakfast Program: Additional Menu Planning Approaches (Final Rule), Federal Register, 65:26904, May 9, 2000	Reinstated traditional food-based menu planning and established an alternate menu-planning approach, thus expanding the menu-planning approaches to five options
2001	No Child Left Behind Act of 2001, P.L. 107-110	Reauthorized the McKinney-Vento Homeless Assistance Act of 1987; provides homeless children with services comparable to those offered to other children in the school, including school nutrition programs; students are automatically enrolled in the program without submission of applications for free or reduced-price meals
2004	Child Nutrition and WIC Reauthorization Act of 2004, P.L. 108-265	Required the Secretary of the Department of Agriculture to issue rules with specific serving recommendations to increase the consumption of foods emphasized by the latest Dietary Guidelines for Americans; mandated that local education agencies develop a local wellness policy to enhance the school nutrition environment; permanently authorized the Fruit and Vegetable Program (which is available to a limited number of states and schools and serves the fruits and vegetables outside the school meal programs); mandated that schools offer fluid milk with a variety of fat contents

Appendix C

Comparison of 1995 and 2005 *Dietary Guidelines for Americans*

This appendix presents a table comparing the 1995 Dietary Guidelines for Americans (HHS/USDA, 1995) with the 2005 Dietary Guidelines for Americans (HHS/USDA, 2005).

TABLE C-1 Comparison of Key Recommendations in the 1995 and 2005 Dietary Guidelines for Americans with Regard to Topics Relevant to the Revision of the Meal Pattern and Nutrition Standard Requirements of the National School Lunch Program and School Breakfast Program

1995 *Dietary Guidelines for Americans*		2005 *Dietary Guidelines for Americans*	
Guideline	Key Context in Text	Focus Area	Key Recommendations
Eat a variety of foods	▪ To obtain the nutrients and other substances needed for good health, vary the foods you eat. ▪ Use foods from the base of the Food Guide Pyramid as the foundation of your meal. ▪ Choose different foods within each food group (grain products, vegetables, fruits, milk and milk products, protein-rich plant foods (beans, nuts), and protein-rich animal foods (lean meat, poultry, fish, and eggs). ▪ Use foods from the base of the Food Guide Pyramid as the foundation of your meal. ▪ Growing children [and] teenage girls … have higher needs for some nutrients (calcium and iron). ▪ Choose lean and low-fat foods and beverages most often.	Adequate nutrients within calorie needs	▪ Consume a variety of nutrient-dense foods and beverages within and among the basic foods groups while choosing foods that limit the intake of saturated fat and *trans fats, cholesterol, added sugars, and salt* ▪ *Meet recommended intakes within energy needs by adopting a balanced eating pattern, such as the U.S. Department of Agriculture (USDA) Food Guide or the Dietary Approaches to Stop Hypertension(DASH) Eating Plan.*
Balance the food you eat with physical activity—maintain or improve your weight	Emphasis is on increasing physical activity, aiming for at least 30 minutes of moderate physical activity on most days of the week, eating foods that are lower in calories, and evaluating body weight.	Weight management	▪ To maintain body weight in a healthy range, balance calories from foods and beverages with calories expended. ▪ To prevent gradual weight gain over time, make small decreases in food and beverage calories and increase physical activity. ▪ *Overweight children: reduce the rate of body weight gain while allowing growth and development. Consult a health care provider before placing a child on a weight-reduction diet.*

Choose a diet with plenty of grain products, vegetables, and fruits	▪ Get most calories from grain products (6–11 servings), vegetables (3–5 servings), and fruits (2–4 servings) each day. ▪ Eat a variety of fiber-containing foods (whole grains and whole-grain products); dry beans, lentils, and peas; and fiber-rich vegetables and fruits).	Food groups to encourage	▪ Consume a sufficient amount of fruits and vegetables while staying within energy needs. *Two cups of fruit and 2½ cups of vegetables per day are recommended for a reference 2,000-calorie intake, with higher or lower amounts depending on the calorie level.* ▪ Choose a variety of fruits and vegetables each day. *In particular, select from all five vegetable subgroups (dark green, orange, legumes, starchy vegetables, and other vegetables) several times a week.* ▪ *Consume whole-grain products often; at least half the grains should be whole grains.* ▪ *Children 2 to 8 years of age should consume 2 cups per day of fat-free or low-fat milk or equivalent milk products. Children 9 years of age and older should consume 3 cups per day of fat-free or low-fat or equivalent milk products.*
Choose a diet low in fat, saturated fat, and cholesterol	▪ Use high-fat foods sparingly. ▪ Choose a diet low in fat (no more than 30 percent of calories from fat). ▪ Choose a diet low in saturated fat (no more than 10 percent of calories from saturated fat). ▪ Choose a diet low in cholesterol (300 mg of cholesterol is identified as the Daily Value or cholesterol on the Nutrition Facts Label of food packages). ▪ Transition to fat limitations applies between ages 2 and 5 years.	Fats	▪ Choose less than 10 percent of calories from saturated fatty acids and *less than 300 mg/day of cholesterol, and keep trans fatty acid consumption as low as possible.* ▪ Keep *total fat intake … to between 25 and 35 percent of calories for children and adolescents 4 to 18 years of age*, with most fats coming from sources of polyunsaturated and monounsaturated fatty acids, such as fish, nuts, and vegetable oils. ▪ When selecting and preparing meat, poultry, dry beans, and milk or milk products, make choices that are lean, low-fat, or fat-free.

Choose a diet moderate in sugars	▪ This helps maintain a nutritious diet and healthy weight. ▪ Sparing use of sugars is indicated for those with low calorie needs. ▪ Avoid excessive snacking. ▪ Regular daily dental hygiene … and an adequate intake of fluoride are suggested.	Carbohydrates	▪ Choose fiber-rich fruits, vegetables, and whole grains *often.* ▪ *Choose and prepare foods and beverages with little added sugars or caloric sweeteners, such as the amounts suggested by the USDA Food Guide and the DASH Eating Plan.* ▪ Reduce the incidence of dental caries by practicing good oral hygiene and *consuming sugar- and starch-containing foods and beverages less often.*
Choose a diet moderate in salt and sodium	▪ Sodium is one of several factors that affect blood pressure. ▪ Most Americans consume more salt than is needed. ▪ Nutrition Facts Labels can help one identify foods that are lower in sodium (2,400 mg of sodium per day is identified as the Daily Value on Nutrition Facts Label).	Sodium and potassium	▪ *Consume less than 2,300 mg of sodium per day.* ▪ *Choose and prepare foods with little salt.* At the same time, *consume potassium-rich foods,* such as fruits and vegetables.

NOTE: Not all text is quoted verbatim. Rewording was necessary, especially when the text touches on a subject without making a specific recommendation. Unless otherwise noted, the text is quoted verbatim. *Italicized font* denotes a new or revised recommendation. If a recommendation for children differs from that for adults, only the recommendation for children is given. Guidelines that pertain specifically to physical activity, food safety, and alcohol consumption were omitted because of lack of relevance to the committee's work.
SOURCES: Derived from HHS/USDA, 1995, 2005.

Appendix D

July 2008 Workshop Agenda

Institute of Medicine
Food and Nutrition Board

Committee to Review National School Lunch and School Breakfast Programs Meal Patterns and Nutrient Standards

INFORMATION-GATHERING OPEN PUBLIC WORKSHOP

The National Academy of Sciences Auditorium
2100 C Street, NW
Washington, DC
July 9, 2008 1:00 p.m.–6:00 p.m.

1:00–1:10 p.m. Welcome and Goals
Virginia Stallings, MD, Chair

1:10–3:15 p.m. SESSION 1: DEVELOPING AND REVISING REQUIREMENTS FOR SCHOOL LUNCH AND BREAKFAST

Perspective on Challenges

1:10–1:20 Food and Nutrition Service, U.S. Department of Agriculture
Jay Hirschman, MPH, CNS, Director, Special Nutrition Staff, Office of Analysis, Nutrition and Evaluation

Perspectives on Possibilities and Approaches

1:20–1:30 National Alliance for Nutrition and Activity
Margo G. Wootan, DSc, Director, Nutrition Policy, Center for Science in the Public Interest

1:30–1:40 Alliance for a Healthier Generation
Kimberly Stitzel, MS, RD, Director of Nutrition and Obesity, Office of Consumer Markets, American Heart Association

1:40–1:50 School Nutrition Association
Katie Wilson, PhD, SNS, School Nutrition Director, Onalaska School District, Wisconsin

1:50–2:00 Hunger and Obesity
Geraldine Henchy, MPH, RD, Director of Nutrition Policy and Early Childhood Programs, Food Research and Action Center
Madeleine Levin, MPH, Senior Policy Analyst, Food Research and Action Center

2:00–2:10 Parental Perspective: National PTA
Kimberly Barnes-O'Connor, PTA Deputy Executive Director, Programs and Public Policy Office

2:10–2:20 Q&A AMONG COMMITTEE AND PRESENTERS

Impact on and Opportunities for the Food Industry

2:20–2:30 Con Agra
Helene Clark, MBA, Director Marketing Health and Wellness, ConAgra Foods Lamb Weston

2:30–2:40 Pierre Foods
Jeanne Harris, Director, School Relations, Pierre Foods

2:40–2:50 General Mills
Adalía Espinosa, Nutrition Scientist II, General Mills: Bell Institute of Health and Nutrition

2:50–3:00 The Schwan Food Company
Sue E. Holbert, RD, LD, Principal Nutrition Scientist, Schwan's Research and Development, Inc.

3:00–3:15 Q&A AMONG COMMITTEE AND PRESENTERS

3:15–3:30 p.m. BREAK

3:30–4:50 p.m. SESSION 2: LESSONS LEARNED FROM STATE AND LOCAL ACTIVITIES: EXPERIENCES AND PRACTICAL CONSIDERATIONS

3:30-3:45 State Experience: North Carolina
Lynn Hoggard, EdD, RD, LDN, FADA, Section Chief, Child Nutrition Services, Division of School Support, North Carolina Department of Public Instruction

3:45-4:00 State Experience: Texas
Fred Higgins, Assistant Commissioner, Texas Department of Agriculture, Food and Nutrition Division

4:00-4:15 Urban Experience: New York City
Ted Spitzer, President, Market Ventures, Inc.

4:15-4:30 Rural Experience: West Virginia
Celeste Peggs, MS, RD, LD, West Virginia Department of Education, Office of Child Nutrition

4:30-4:50 Q&A AMONG COMMITTEE AND PRESENTERS

4:50–5:00 p.m. BREAK

5:00–6:00 PUBLIC COMMENTS (5 MINUTES EACH)
American Academy of Pediatrics (*Cindy Pellegrini*)
Sunkist Taylor LLC (*Rick Harris*)
International Dairy Foods Association (*Michelle Albee Matto*)
National Dairy Council (*Jill Nicholls*)
American Dietetic Association (*Martin M. Yadrick*)
United Egg Producers (*Howard Magwire*)
U.S. Apple Association (*Diane C. Kurrle*)
ARAMARK Education (*Linda Sceurman*)
Action for Healthy Kids (*Vanessa Cavallaro*)

Appendix E

Critical Issues for Consideration by the Committee[1]

There are a number of important issues on which USDA particularly seeks guidance. In the descriptions below, we have raised a number of questions and concerns, as well as tentative policy concepts for IOM's critical review. These are intended to clarify the scope of the committee's charge, but not to constrain or pre-determine its recommendations. We also ask the committee to consider such operational factors as market conditions, impacts on student acceptability of meals, and the decision to participate in the program, in making recommendations in each of these areas.

Calorie requirements:
Since the establishment of the school meal programs, the dietary concerns for children have shifted from preventing hunger and nutritional deficiencies to recognizing the increase of childhood overweight/obesity rates while enhancing cognitive performance and academic achievement. FNS requests that the committee provide recommendations for calorie levels in consideration of the best scientific information available (including the DRIs) that reflect the diversity of energy needs in today's school children. FNS would like the IOM committee to provide minimum calorie requirements, and consider also recommending maximum calorie levels for reimbursable meals that take into consideration age-grade groupings.

Age-grade groups:
The NSLP and SBP provide meals for children age two and older (generally, under 21). The meal programs group children according to age-grade and establish meal patterns with minimum portion sizes and servings to help menu planners design meals that are age-appropriate and meet the diverse nutritional needs of school children. Nutrient and calorie requirements are also determined for each age-grade groups. In light of the childhood obesity trend, FNS is concerned that school meals provide age-appropriate portion sizes and promote the development of healthy eating behaviors. We request that the committee recommend age-grade groups that are consistent for all menu planning approaches and reflect the stages of growth and development in children and adolescents.

[1] Provided by USDA to the committee.

School grade structures and meal service operations must be considered to ensure that age-grade group recommendations can be successfully implemented. Specifically, in the NSLP, some schools currently use a single age-grade group to plan meals for children and adolescents. The Department is concerned that for lunch meals intended to provide ⅓ of the RDAs without providing excessive calories, this practice may result in meals that fail to meet the nutritional needs of either group. While the same may be true for SBP, where the meals are intended to provide 1/4 of the RDAs, FNS recognizes that there are different operational constraints. In the SBP, children typically participate as they arrive at school, rather than by grade level or other service schedule that would be common in lunch. The single age-grade group currently allowed for SBP menu planning is intended to provide flexibility to meet the needs of the SBP foodservice operation. Also of note, many schools have implemented alternative methods of delivering meals to promote student participation, such as Breakfast in the Classroom or Grab-and-Go Breakfasts. FNS requests that the committee consider the potential impacts that age-grade group requirements may have on the unique aspects of NSLP and SBP meal service, operations, and participation.

Nutrient standards:
FNS requests that in addition to the current required nutrients, the IOM committee consider the DGA recommendations to minimize *trans* fats, as well as the intake recommendations for sodium, cholesterol, and fiber, which currently do not have quantitative standards in the school meal programs. Program operators are currently required to reduce sodium and cholesterol levels and to increase fibers levels. Monitoring these nutrients has been facilitated by the Nutrition Labeling and Education Act requirement that sodium, cholesterol, and fiber amounts be included on food labels and product specifications. Furthermore, *trans* fats information is now required to be included on the Nutrition Facts label and on product specifications, which would facilitate the ability of Program operators and administrators to monitor compliance with the *trans* fats recommendation.

Total fat:
The DGA recommendation for fat is to keep total fat intake between 30 to 35 percent of calories for children 2 to 3 years of age and between 25 to 35 percent of calories daily for children and adolescents 4 to 18 years of age. It should be noted that breakfast meals are often relatively low in fat (below 25 percent). The fat recommendation for each of the meals, in addition to the total daily fat range, should be considered in this process.

Available nutrient information:
Program operators and administrators rely in part on nutrition information provided by food labels and product specifications to plan and assess menus that meet the required nutrient levels. FNS is concerned that establishing requirements for nutrients that are not required to be listed on food labels and product specifications by the Nutrition Labeling and Education Act (NLEA, P.L. 101-535), such as the nutrients of concern for children including potassium, magnesium, and vitamin E, would be a burden to Program operators and administrators. FNS requests that nutrient standard recommendations take into consideration the availability of nutrient information on food labels and product specifications.

Sodium standard:

It is well-recognized that the current intake of sodium for most individuals in the U.S., including school-age children, greatly exceeds the DGA recommendation to consume less than 2300 milligrams (mg) of sodium per day. FNS has encouraged schools to reduce sodium in the NSLP and SBP since the implementation of the School Meals Initiative (SMI) in 1995; however, the School Nutrition Dietary Assessment Studies (SNDA I - III) consistently indicate that the efforts since 1995 have not resulted in any significant reduction of sodium levels in school meals, on average.

FNS is concerned that the challenge of reducing sodium levels in school meals extends beyond the efforts of Program operators and administrators alone. At present, sodium is a common addition to processed foods and convenience items which are commonly used in school meal programs to save time and reduce labor costs. Additionally, the availability of high sodium foods at home, at restaurants, and at other locations in and outside of the school meals programs has resulted in a taste preference for salty foods which impacts student acceptability of school meals and Program participation. Furthermore, it takes time to change children's taste preferences and for industry to respond to a need for low-sodium products in schools and the general market.

The USDA requests that the committee consider student acceptability, Program participation, and market conditions when making recommendations for sodium levels in school meals. Additionally, the Department requests that the committee consider a recommendation that would allow for a progressive or gradual reduction of sodium levels in school meals, such as interim targets, to ultimately meet a standard based on the DGA recommendation over a realistic period of time without adversely affecting program participation.

Vitamin A standard:

Current regulations require that school meals meet minimum levels of vitamin A expressed in Retinol Equivalents (RE), as specified in the 1989 RDAs. The nutrition facts panel on food products provides vitamin A levels in International Units (IU). The most recent DRI standards for vitamin A are quantified in Retinol Activity Equivalents (RAE). FNS is concerned that there is no direct conversion from the DRI recommendations in RAE to IU. FNS requests that the committee recommend a vitamin A standard that addresses the fact that Program operators and administrators rely both on values in nutrient analysis software (which may be in RAE, RE and/or IU) and on food labels and product specifications that quantify vitamin A in IU (i.e., percent of Daily Value in International Units). FNS recognizes that a conversion from levels expressed in RAE to IU may need to be based on representation of a mixed diet for school-aged children.

Menu planning approaches:

FNS would like the committee to examine the adequacy of the current menu planning approaches in meeting the applicable DRIs and DGAs. We are concerned that the structure of the current menu planning approaches, such as the Traditional FBMP and NSMP, may no longer be adequate to provide school meals that reflect the 2005 DGAs. Furthermore, FNS would like recommendations for a single food-based menu planning and a single nutrient standard menu planning approach. FNS requests that the IOM recommendations result in age-appropriate meals and reflect the applicable DRIs and 2005 DGAs under any menu planning approach.

Fruit, vegetables, whole grains and low-fat/fat-free milk products:
The Child Nutrition and WIC Reauthorization Act of 2004 amended the NSLA to require increased consumption of foods that are specifically recommended in the most recent DGAs. FNS is requesting recommendations to increase the availability of the food groups encouraged by the 2005 DGAs. FNS wishes to apply requirements for these food groups to ensure that all students in the NSLP and SBP have access to adequate amounts of these recommended foods, regardless of the menu planning approach used by their school foodservice authority.

Current NSLP regulations require that minimum servings of fruits and/or vegetables, fluid milk, and whole grain or enriched sources of grains/breads be offered daily in the food-based menu planning approaches. In the nutrient standard menu planning approaches, fluid milk is the only required food item to be offered and minimum serving requirements are not established. Under all menu planning approaches, whole grains are encouraged but not required. Additionally, all schools must provide a variety of fluid milk types (a minimum of two); regulations do not place restrictions on offering any milk-fat or flavored varieties.

In the SBP, meal patterns and menu structures have been designed to provide schools with flexibility to provide meals that reflect a typical breakfast meal and avoid unnecessary burden on school foodservice operations. FNS requests that the committee consider such differences between NSLP and SBP meal service operations when making recommendations to increase the food groups encouraged by the 2005 DGAs in the FBMP breakfast meal pattern and the NSMP menu structure.

Special considerations for whole grains:

- In order to incorporate whole grains into the menus, schools must be able to accurately identify a creditable whole-grain product. An issue for FNS is helping schools easily identify whole grain products that provide a significant level of whole grains. At this time, the FDA has not published a definition of a whole-grain product, or a whole-grain serving. USDA wishes to establish a consistent definition for all the FNS Special Nutrition Programs (including NSLP, SBP, Child and Adult Care Food Program, the Summer Food Service Program (SFSP), WIC, and the FNS commodity programs).

Special considerations for fluid milk:

- The NSLA and program regulations require that lunches include fluid milk and allow fluid milk in a variety of fat contents and flavors. Fluid milk may not be substituted by another beverage or dairy product, except when a disability precludes milk consumption.[2] Under the FBMP approaches, a minimum of eight fluid ounces is required for school-age

[2] Current regulations require milk substitutions for students with disabilities when supported by a statement from a physician. Substitutions for students with special or other dietary needs are optional and must be supported by a statement from a medical authority such as a nurse. USDA issued a proposal on November 6, 2006 to allow schools to accept a parent statement in lieu of a statement from a medical authority. The proposed rule also specified nutrient standards for the non-dairy milk substitutes offered to students with special or other dietary needs. A final rule is in development.

children and a minimum of six fluid ounces is required for preschoolers. No minimum quantity is required under the NSMP approaches. Since calcium is a nutrient of concern for children and milk is a primary food source of nutrients for children, FNS is seeking recommendations to implement the recommendations of the DGAs and DRIs. When considering this, the IOM expert committee should also address concerns that offering different quantity for the various age-grade groups in the NSLP and SBP may be operationally difficult to implement at the local school level due to procurement logistics and economies of scale.

Meat/Meat Alternate:

The current meat/meat alternate requirements in the NSLP meal patterns exceed the recommended quantities in the USDA Food Guide, the food pattern that illustrates the recommendations of the DGAs. The School Nutrition Dietary Assessment (SNDA) studies show that current meal patterns require more than adequate amounts of meat/meat alternate to meet the nutritional (protein and iron) needs of children and adolescents. There may be adjustments to existing meat/meat alternate requirements that could help schools limit food costs while still meeting the nutritional needs of participants. Schools could meet the meat/meat alternate requirement over the course of the week as long as a minimum serving of meat/meat alternate is offered daily. Consistent with the DGAs, schools should offer low-fat, lean meat/meal alternates to help children limit the intakes of saturated fat, total fat, and cholesterol. In addition, there is public interest in incorporating nutrient-dense meat alternatives such as soy-based products in the NSLP.

Offer versus Serve:

The IOM committee may need to be aware of Offer versus Serve, a statutory requirement intended to reduce plate waste in the lunch program. The NSLA requires that high school students be allowed to decline foods they do not intend to eat. Offer versus Serve may be implemented at lower grades at the option of the local school district. Program regulations require that students select at least three of the five food items offered in a food-based menu. For nutrient-based menus, the regulations require that students select the entrée. If three items are offered, students may decline one; if four or more items are offered, students may decline two.

Attainable recommendations:

The majority of schools prepare meals on-site with a small staff and restricted budget. Food purchasing, planning, preparation and service are often carried out by employees with no formal food service or management training. Changes to the meal patterns and nutrition standards must be feasible for school foodservice operators, and should not jeopardize student and school participation in the meal programs. To ensure that the combined set of recommendations are attainable, the Department requests IOM to include in the report separately for NSLP and SBP a set of four- week cycle menus for each of the recommended age groups that meet all recommendations, are relatively cost neutral and would not likely have an adverse effect on program participation.

Appendix F

Selected Evaluations of School Meal Programs

The following table presents USDA-funded large-scale studies that evaluate the school meal programs and may be relevant to updating the Nutrition Standards and Meal Requirements.

TABLE F-1 Selected Evaluations of School Meal Programs of Potential Relevance to Updating the Nutrition Standards and Meal Requirements

Date of Publication	Evaluation	Reference or Link to Report
1983	National Evaluation of School Nutrition Programs	Wellisch et al., 1983
October 1993	School Nutrition Dietary Assessment Study I	Summary of Findings: http://www.fns.usda.gov/OANE/menu/Published/CNP/FILES/SNDA-Sum.pdf
October 1994	School Lunch and Breakfast Cost Study I	Summary of Findings: http://www.fns.usda.gov/OANE/menu/Published/CNP/FILES/Lunch_BreakfastCostSum.pdf
February 1997	Evaluation of the Nutrient Standard Menu Planning Demonstration: Findings from the Formative Evaluation	Summary of Findings: http://www.fns.usda.gov/OANE/menu/Published/CNP/FILES/FORMSUM.htm
August 1998	Eating Breakfast: Effects of the School Breakfast Program	Executive Summary: http://www.fns.usda.gov/OANE/menu/Published/CNP/FILES/SBPEXSUM.htm
August 1998	Nutrient Standard Menu Planning Evaluation Summary	Summary of Findings: http://www.fns.usda.gov/OANE/menu/Published/CNP/FILES/nsmpdem.pdf
September 1998	School Food Purchase Study	Executive Summary: http://www.fns.usda.gov/OANE/menu/Published/CNP/FILES/SFPS-Execsum.pdf
July 1999	Team Nutrition Pilot Study	Executive Summary: http://www.fns.usda.gov/OANE/menu/Published/CNP/FILES/tn2execsum.pdf
October 2000	School Meal Initiative Implementation Study: Year 1 Report	Executive Summary: http://www.fns.usda.gov/OANE/menu/Published/CNP/FILES/SMIexecsum.htm
January 2001	Children's Diets in the Mid-1990s (Continuing Survey of Food Intakes by Individuals 1994–1996 data)	Executive Summary: http://www.fns.usda.gov/OANE/menu/Published/CNP/FILES/ChilDietsum.htm
April 2001	School Nutrition Dietary Assessment Study II	Executive Summary: http://www.fns.usda.gov/OANE/menu/Published/CNP/FILES/SNDAIIfindsum.htm

July 2001	School Meal Initiative Implementation Study: Year 2 Report	Executive Summary: http://www.fns.usda.gov/OANE/menu/Published/CNP/FILES/SMIYear2.htm
March 2002	Plate Waste in School Nutrition Programs: Final Report to Congress	Report: http://www.ers.usda.gov/publications/efan02009/efan02009.pdf
April 2002	School Lunch Salad Bars	Executive Summary: http://www.fns.usda.gov/OANE/menu/Published/CNP/FILES/SaladBars.htm
May 2002	Availability of Fresh Produce in Nutrition Assistance Programs	Executive Summary: http://www.fns.usda.gov/OANE/menu/Published/CNP/FILES/FVSummary.htm
June 2002	School Meal Initiative Implementation Study: Year 3 and Final Report	Executive Summary: http://www.fns.usda.gov/OANE/menu/Published/CNP/FILES/SMIYear3.htm
October 2002	Evaluation of the School Breakfast Program Pilot Project: Findings from the First Year of Implementation	Executive Summary: http://www.fns.usda.gov/OANE/menu/Published/CNP/FILES/breakfastyr1.htm
December 2004	Evaluation of the School Breakfast Program Pilot Project: Final Report	Executive Summary: http://www.fns.usda.gov/OANE/menu/Published/CNP/FILES/SBPPExecSum.pdf
November 2007	School Nutrition Dietary Assessment Study III	Executive Summary: http://www.fns.usda.gov/OANE/menu/Published/CNP/FILES/SNDAIII-Vol1ExecSum.pdf
April 2008	School Lunch and Breakfast Cost Study II	Executive Summary: http://www.fns.usda.gov/OANE/menu/Published/CNP/FILES/MealCostStudyExecSum.pdf

Appendix G

Current Standards for Food-Based Menu Planning Approach

The following tables include the food components and the amounts for the food-based menu planning approaches for lunch and breakfast *as offered* and *as served.*

TABLE G-1 Reimbursable Lunch: Standards for Food Components *as Offered* and *as Served*

As Offered	As Served
• One fluid milk • One meat/meat alternate • Two vegetable/fruit • One grain/bread *(Total= five items)*	Senior high school level: students must select three of the five items Grades below senior high school level[a]: students must select either three or four of the five items

[a]Offer versus serve is optional below the senior high school level.
SOURCE: USDA, 2007b.

TABLE G-2 Reimbursable Lunch: Standards for Amounts of Food Items for Age-Grade Groups

	Traditional Approach				Enhanced Approach			
	Minimum Requirements			Optional,	Minimum Requirements			Optional,
Food Component or food item	Preschool	Grades K–3	Grades 4–12[a]	Grades 7–12	Preschool	Grades K–6	Grades 7–12	Grades K–3
Fluid milk (as a beverage)	6 fluid oz	8 fluid oz	8 fluid oz	8 fluid oz	6 fluid oz	8 fluid oz	8 fluid oz	8 fluid oz
Meat/meat alternate								
Lean meat, poultry, or fish	1½ oz	1½ oz	2 oz	3 oz	1½ oz	2 oz	2 oz	1½ oz
Alternate Protein Products[b]	1½ oz	1½ oz	2 oz	3 oz	1½ oz	2 oz	2 oz	1½ oz
Cheese	1½ oz	1½ oz	2 oz	3 oz	1½ oz	2 oz	2 oz	1½ oz
Large egg	¾	¾	1	1 ½	¾	1	1	¾
Cooked dry beans or peas	⅜ cup	⅜ cup	½ cup	¾ cup	⅜ cup	½ cup	½ cup	⅜ cup
Peanut butter, other nuts, or seed butters	3 tbsp	3 tbsp	4 tbsp	6 tbsp	3 tbsp	4 tbsp	4 tbsp	3 tbsp
Yogurt, plain or flavored, unsweetened or sweetened	6 oz or ¾ cup	6 oz or ¾ cup	8 oz or 1 cup	12 oz or 1½ cups	6 oz or ¾ cup	8 oz or 1 cup	8 oz or 1 cup	6 oz or ¾ cup

	Traditional				Enhanced			
	Minimum Requirements				Minimum Requirements			
Food component or food item	Preschool	Grades K–3	Grades 4–12[a]	Optional, Grades 7–12	Preschool	Grades K–6	Grades 7–12	Optional, Grades K–3
Peanuts, soy nuts, tree nuts, or seeds[c,d]	¾ oz	¾ oz	1 oz	1½ oz	¾ oz	1 oz	1 oz	¾ oz
Vegetable/fruit	½ cup	½ cup	¾ cup	¾ cup	½ cup	¾ cup[e]	1 cup	¾ cup
Grain/bread[f]	8 servings per week	8 servings per week	8 servings per week	10 servings per week	8 servings per week	12 servings per week	15 servings per week	10 servings per week

NOTE: K = kindergarten; oz = ounce; tbsp = tablespoon.

[a]The school food authority or school always has the option of serving the grades 4–12 age-grade groups for all students in the school district or school under the traditional food-based approach for lunch.

[b]Examples of Alternate Protein Products include soy flours, soy concentrates, soy isolates, whey protein concentrate, whey protein isolates, and casein.

[c]As listed in the program guidance or an equivalent quantity of any combination of the meats/meat alternates listed above.

[d]May be used to meet no more than 50 percent of the requirement and must be used in combination with any of the meats/meat alternates listed above. The amounts listed in the table are 50 percent of the requirement. (1 ounce of nuts or seeds = 1 ounce of cooked lean meat, poultry, or fish.)

[e]Also required to have an extra 1/2 cup over a week. For the purpose of this table, a week equals 5 days.

[f]Must be enriched with whole grain. Minimum of one serving per day. A serving is a slice of bread or an equivalent serving of biscuits, rolls, etc., or 1/2 cup of cooked rice, macaroni, noodles, other pasta products, or cereal grains.

SOURCE: Derived from USDA, 2000b, with additional information from USDA, 2007b.

TABLE G-3 Reimbursable Breakfast: Standards for Food Components *as Offered* and *as Served*[a]

As Offered	As Served
• One fluid milk • One vegetable/fruit • Two meat/meat alternate; two grain/bread; or one meat/meat alternate and one grain/bread *(Total=four items)*	Students may decline a maximum of one of the four items

[a]Offer versus serve for breakfast is optional at all grade levels.
SOURCE: USDA, 2007b.

TABLE G-4 Reimbursable Breakfast: Standards for Amounts of Food Items for Age-Grade Groups

	Traditional Approach		Enhanced Approach		
	Minimum Requirements		Minimum Requirements		
Food Component or Food Item	Preschool	Grades K–12	Preschool	Grades K–12	Optional, Grades 7–12
Fluid milk (as a beverage, on cereal, or both)	6 fluid oz	8 fluid oz	6 fluid oz	8 fluid oz	8 fluid oz
Meat/meat alternate					
Lean meat, poultry, or fish	½ oz	1 oz	½ oz	1 oz	1 oz
Alternate Protein Products[a]	½ oz	1 oz	½ oz	1 oz	1 oz
Cheese	½ oz	1 oz	½ oz	1 oz	1 oz
Large egg	½	½	½	½	½
Cooked dry beans or peas	2 tbsp	4 tbsp	2 tbsp	4 tbsp	4 tbsp
Peanut butter, other nut, or seed butters	1 tbsp	2 tbsp	1 tbsp	2 tbsp	2 tbsp
Yogurt, plain or flavored, unsweetened or sweetened	2 oz or ¼ cup	4 oz or ½ cup	2 oz or ¼ cup	4 oz or ½ cup	4 oz or ½ cup
Peanuts, soy nuts, tree nuts, or seeds[b]	½ oz	1 oz	½ oz	1 oz	1 oz

	Traditional		Enhanced		
	Minimum Requirements		Minimum Requirements		
Food Component or Food Item	Preschool	Grades K–12	Preschool	Grades K–12	Optional, Grades 7–12
Vegetable/fruit	½ cup	½ cup	½ cup	½ cup	½ cup
Grain/bread					
Whole-grain or enriched bread	½ slice	1 slice	½ slice	1 slice	1 slice
Whole-grain or enriched biscuit, roll, muffin, etc.	½ serving	1 serving	½ serving	1 serving	1 serving
Whole-grain, enriched, or fortified cereal	⅓ cup or ½oz	¾ cup or 1 oz	⅓ cup or ½ oz	¾ cup or 1 oz	¾ cup or 1 oz[c]

NOTE: K = kindergarten; oz = ounce; tbsp = tablespoon.

[a]Examples of Alternate Protein Products include soy flours, soy concentrates, soy isolates, whey protein concentrate, whey protein isolates, and casein.

[b]No more than 1 ounce of nuts and/or seeds may be served in any one breakfast.

[c]Plus one additional serving of any of the grains/breads listed above.

SOURCE: Derived from USDA, 2008f, with additional information from USDA, 2007b.

Appendix H

Current Standards for Nutrient-Based Menu Planning Approach

The following tables include the menu items and the amounts for the nutrient-based menu planning approaches for lunch and breakfast *as offered* and *as served.*

TABLE H-1 Reimbursable Lunch and Breakfast: Standards for Menu Items *as Offered* and *as Served*

	As Offered	As Served
Lunch[a]	Schools must offer at least 3 menu items: • Fluid milk • Entrée • Side dish	• If 3 items are offered, students may decline 1 • If 4 or more items are offered, students may decline 2 • Students must select an entrée
Breakfast[b]	Schools must offer at least 3 menu items: • Fluid milk (served as a beverage) • 2 additional menu items	• Student may decline only 1 item, regardless of the number of items offered

[a]Offer versus serve (OVS) is optional in grades below senior high level.
[b]OVS for breakfast is optional at all grade levels.

TABLE H-2 Reimbursable Lunch and Breakfast: Standards for 5-Day Average Amounts of the Key Nutrients for Age-Grade Groups

	Lunch				Breakfast		
	Minimum Requirements			Optional	Minimum Requirements		Optional
	Preschool	K-6	Grades 7-12	K-3	Preschool	K-12	Grades 7-12
Calories	517	664	825	633	388	554	618
Fat (% of calories)	≤30%	≤30%	≤30%	≤30%	≤30%	≤30%	≤30%
Saturated Fat (% of calories)	<10%	<10%	<10%	<10%	<10%	<10%	<10%
Protein (g)	7	10	16	9	5	10	12
Calcium (mg)	267	286	400	267	200	257	300
Iron (mg)	3.3	3.5	4.5	3.3	2.5	3.0	3.4
Vitamin A (RAE)	150	224	300	200	113	197	225
Vitamin C (mg)	14	15	18	15	11	13	14

NOTE: g = grams; K = kindergarten; mg = milligrams; RAE = retinol activity equivalent.
SOURCE: Derived from USDA, 2000b, 2008f.

Appendix I

Data Sources and Study Methodology: SNDA-III and 2008 Diet Quality Report[1]

THIRD SCHOOL NUTRITION DIETARY ASSESSMENT STUDY

Sample Design and Sampling

The Third School Nutrition Dietary Assessment Study (SNDA-III) (USDA, 2007a) sample was designed to be representative of all public school food authorities (SFAs) participating in the NSLP, schools in those SFAs, and students in grades 1–12 in those schools. The SFAs sampled were selected with probability proportional to size (PPS; the measure of size was the student enrollment). Within each SFA, one elementary school, one middle school, and one high school were selected with PPS, in general (in districts without all three levels, the procedures were adjusted). The students within the schools were randomly sampled. In addition, a supplemental sample of SFAs and schools from which no student-level data were collected was included to provide additional precision for school-level estimates. If any SFAs, schools, or students declined to participate in the data collection effort, they were replaced by randomly chosen substitutes.

SFAs eligible for the sample were public SFAs that were located in the continental United States and that did not serve either residential facilities or solely special education students. The schools within these SFAs were eligible unless they served only prekindergarten, kindergarten, or special education students. All students in grades 1–12 in these schools except those in self-contained special education classes were eligible to participate. Students in self-contained special education classes were omitted from the study because of concerns about their ability to complete the recall interview.

A total of 130 SFAs participated in the study. School-level data were collected from 398 schools in these SFAs. Student-level data were collected onsite from students in a random subset of 287 schools in 94 SFAs. About 8 students per school completed both a dietary recall and had a parent complete an interview, the criteria for being included in the analysis sample; 2,314 students met those criteria.

[1]Sources: the third School Nutrition Dietary Assessment (USDA, 2007a) and *Diet Quality of American School-Age Children by School Lunch Participation Status*: data from the National Health and Nutrition Examination Survey, 1999–2004 (USDA, 2008l).

Collection and Analysis of Dietary Recall Data

SNDA-III dietary recalls were collected by using a modified version of the Automated Multiple Pass Method software (version 2.3, 2003, Agricultural Research Service, Food Surveys Research Group, Beltsville, MD), which has been used to collect data for the for National Health and Nutrition Examination Survey (NHANES) since 2003. Children in middle and high schools were interviewed in the morning and reported the previous day's intake (from midnight to midnight). Because young children tend to have difficulty recalling their intakes, interviews with young children were completed in two parts and with parental assistance. These children were first interviewed during the school day, after lunch if possible, and were asked to report everything that they had consumed that day since awakening. They were then interviewed a second time to report their intakes for the rest of the 24-hour period. The second interviews were conducted on the next day, if possible, and were conducted no more than 48 hours after the first interview. Parents attended the second in-person interviews and were asked to help their children recall and describe the foods and beverages consumed.

The SurveyNet coding system (version 3.14, 2004, Agricultural Research Service, U.S. Department of Agriculture [USDA], Beltsville, MD) was used to link each item reported in the 24-hour recalls to the Food and Nutrient Database for Dietary Studies (FNDDS; version 1.0, 2004, Agricultural Research Service, Food Surveys Research Group, Beltsville, MD). Subsequently, for foods and beverages that were obtained at school from reimbursable meal sources and that were reported on school menus, FNDDS nutrient values were replaced with nutrient values from the analysis of the school menus (USDA, 2007a). This step ensured that foods provided as part of the National School Lunch Program and the School Breakfast Program were represented in the analysis as accurately as possible. For example, rather than hamburgers or cheese pizzas obtained at school being consistently represented by the default values available in the nutrient database, the nutrient value of the hamburgers and pizzas actually served in each child's school were used. Thus, if a school purchased extra-lean hamburger patties or pizzas made with less or low-fat cheese, this was reflected in the 24-hour recall data.

2008 DIET QUALITY REPORT

All tabulations for the *Diet Quality of American School-Age Children by School Lunch Participation Status* (referred to as the 2008 Diet Quality Report) are based on data from NHANES 1999–2004, analyzed alone or in conjunction with data from the MyPyramid Equivalents Database.

NHANES is conducted by the National Center for Health Statistics (NCHS), which is part of the Centers for Disease Control and Prevention. NHANES has been conducted on a periodic basis since 1971. Beginning in 1999, NHANES has been a continuous annual survey and data are released in public data files every 2 years (e.g., 1999–2000, 2001–2002, and 2003–2004). NCHS recommends that data from two or more 2-year cycles of the continuous NHANES be combined to increase the sample size and produce estimates with greater statistical reliabilities. Most of the tabulations presented in this report are based on three 2-year cycles of NHANES data (1999–2004) and are based on data from the following NHANES data files:

- Body Measures (BMX);
- Demographics (DEMO);

- Dietary Interview Individual Food Files (DRXIFF); and
- Dietary Interview, Total Nutrient Intakes (DRXTOT).

The analysis sample for estimates of usual nutrient intakes included 3,546 children who were enrolled in school and completed a 24-hour recall during NHANES 1999–2004 on a weekday when school was in session.[2,3] Estimates of MyPyramid food intakes are based on a sample of 2,597 children who completed a 24-hour recall under similar circumstances during NHANES 1999–2002.[4]

---

[2]The sample was limited in this manner to capture dietary behavior among children attending school. NHANES did not begin collecting data on whether a child attended school on the day of the dietary recall until 2003. For the other years, school calendars collected from counties represented in the NHANES sample were used to identify the calendar dates when school was likely to be in session. However, some children may not actually have been in school on the day of the recall because of illness, the children were absent for another reason, the school had a snow day, or the school was closed for some other reason.

[3]NHANES did not begin collecting the second 24-hour recall needed to estimate usual energy and nutrient intake distributions until the 2003 data collection cycle. The second recall is attempted with all respondents and is done by telephone. In 2003–2004, 87 percent of the NHANES respondents who completed the first 24-hour call completed the second recall. The usual energy and nutrient intake distributions reported in the 2008 Diet Quality Report are based on single 24-hour recalls reported in NHANES 1999–2004 and the second 24-hour recalls reported in NHANES 2003–2004.

[4]Children in the NHANES 2003–2004 sample were not included in these tabulations because a companion database used to estimate food intakes (the MyPyramid Equivalents Database for USDA Food Codes [version 1.0; USDA, 2006a]) provides data only for NHANES 1999–2000 and 2001–2002.

Appendix J

MyPyramid Calorie Levels and Food Intake Patterns

TABLE J-1 MyPyramid Food Intake Pattern Calorie Levels

Males				Females			
	Activity Level				Activity Level		
Age (yr)	Sedentary	Moderately Active	Active	Age (yr)	Sedentary	Moderately Active	Active
2	1,000	1,000	1,000	2	1,000	1,000	1,000
3	1,000	1,000	1,400	3	1,000	1,200	1,400
4	1,200	1,400	1,600	4	1,200	1,400	1,400
5	1,200	1,400	1,600	5	1,200	1,400	1,600
6	1,400	1,600	1,800	6	1,200	1,400	1,600
7	1,400	1,600	1,800	7	1,200	1,600	1,800
8	1,400	1,600	2,000	8	1,400	1,600	1,800
9	1,600	1,800	2,000	9	1,400	1,600	1,800
10	1,600	1,800	2,200	10	1,400	1,800	2,000
11	1,800	2,000	2,200	11	1,600	1,800	2,000
12	1,800	2,200	2,400	12	1,600	2,000	2,200
13	2,000	2,200	2,600	13	1,600	2,000	2,200
14	2,000	2,400	2,800	14	1,800	2,000	2,400
15	2,200	2,600	3,000	15	1,800	2,000	2,400
16	2,400	2,800	3,200	16	1,800	2,000	2,400
17	2,400	2,800	3,200	17	1,800	2,000	2,400
18	2,400	2,800	3,200	18	1,800	2,000	2,400

NOTE: Calorie levels are based on the Estimated Energy Requirements, and activity levels are from the Institute of Medicine report *Dietary Reference Intakes for Energy, Carbohydrate, Fiber, Fat, Fatty Acids, Cholesterol, Protein, and Amino Acids (Macronutrients)* (IOM, 2002/2005). sedentary = less than 30 minutes a day of moderate physical activity, in addition to daily activities; moderately active = at least 30 minutes up to 60 minutes a day of moderate physical activity, in addition to daily activities; active = 60 or more minutes a day of moderate physical activity, in addition to daily activities.

TABLE J-2 MyPyramid Food Intake Patterns

	Intake Pattern for the Following Calorie Level:											
Food	1,000	1,200	1,400	1,600	1,800	2,000	2,200	2,400	2,600	2,800	3,000	3,200
Fruits	1 cup	1 cup	1.5 cups	1.5 cups	1.5 cups	2 cups	2 cups	2 cups	2 cups	2.5 cups	2.5 cups	2.5 cups
Vegetables	1 cup	1.5 cups	1.5 cups	2 cups	2.5 cups	2.5 cups	3 cups	3 cups	3.5 cups	3.5 cups	4 cups	4 cups
Dark green vegetables	1 c/wk	1.5 c/wk	1.5 c/wk	2 c/wk	3 c/wk	3 c/wk	3 c/wk	3 c/wk	3 c/wk	3 c/wk	3 c/wk	3 c/wk
Orange vegetables	0.5 c/wk	1 c/wk	1 c/wk	1.5 c/wk	2 c/wk	2 c/wk	2 c/wk	2 c/wk	2.5 c/wk	2.5 c/wk	2.5 c/wk	2.5 c/wk
Legumes	0.5 c/wk	1 c/wk	1 c/wk	2.5 c/wk	3 c/wk	3 c/wk	3 c/wk	3 c/wk	3.5 c/wk	3.5 c/wk	3.5 c/wk	3.5 c/wk
Starchy vegetables	1.5 c/wk	2.5 c/wk	2.5 c/wk	2.5 c/wk	3 c/wk	3 c/wk	6 c/wk	6 c/wk	7 c/wk	7 c/wk	9 c/wk	9 c/wk
Other vegetables	3.5 c/wk	4.5 c/wk	4.5 c/wk	5.5 c/wk	6.5 c/wk	6.5 c/wk	7 c/wk	7 c/wk	8.5 c/wk	8.5 c/wk	10 c/wk	10 c/wk
Grains[a]	3 oz eq	4 oz eq	5 oz eq	5 oz eq	6 oz eq	6 oz eq	7 oz eq	8 oz eq	9 oz eq	10 oz eq	10 oz eq	10 oz eq
Meats and beans	2 oz eq	3 oz eq	4 oz eq	5 oz eq	5 oz eq	5.5 oz eq	6 oz eq	6.5 oz eq	6.5 oz eq	7 oz eq	7 oz eq	7 oz eq
Milk	2 cups	2 cups	2 cups	3 cups	3 cups	3 cups	3 cups	3 cups	3 cups	3 cups	3 cups	3 cups
Oils	3 tsp	4 tsp	4 tsp	5 tsp	5 tsp	6 tsp	6 tsp	7 tsp	8 tsp	8 tsp	10 tsp	11 tsp
Discretionary calorie allowance	165	171	171	132	195	267	290	362	410	426	512	648

NOTE: c/wk = cups per week; oz eq = ounce equivalent; tsp = teaspoon.

[a]Grains should include a minimum of three 1-ounce servings of whole grains, and for those with daily food intakes of greater than 1,600 calories, half of grains should be whole grains.

SOURCE: USDA, 2005b.

Appendix K

Dietary Reference Intakes for Individuals Ages 4 Through 18 Years, Including Those Who Are Pregnant or Lactating

The following tables include the Dietary Reference Intakes (DRIs) for schoolchildren.

TABLE K-1 DRIs: Estimated Average Requirements for Groups

Life-Stage Group	CHO (g/d)	Protein (g/d)	Vitamin A (μg/d)[a]	Vitamin C (mg/d)	Vitamin E (mg/d)[b]	Thiamin (mg/d)	Riboflavin (mg/d)	Niacin (mg/d)[c]	Vitamin B_6 (mg/d)	Folate (μg/d)[d]	Vitamin B_{12} (μg/d)	Copper (μg/d)	Iodine (μg/d)	Iron (mg/d)	Magnesium (mg/d)	Molybdenum (μg/d)	Phosphorus (mg/d)	Selenium (μg/d)	Zinc (mg/d)
Children																			
4–8 yr	100	15	275	22	6	0.5	0.5	6	0.5	160	1.0	340	65	4.1	110	17	405	23	4.0
Males																			
9–13 yr	100	27	445	39	9	0.7	0.8	9	0.8	250	1.5	540	73	5.9	200	26	1,055	35	7.0
14–18 yr	100	44	630	63	12	1.0	1.1	12	1.1	330	2.0	685	95	7.7	340	33	1,055	45	8.5
Females																			
9–13 yr	100	28	420	39	9	0.7	0.8	9	0.8	250	1.5	540	73	5.7	200	26	1,055	35	7.0
14–18 yr	100	38	485	56	12	0.9	0.9	11	1.0	330	2.0	685	95	7.9	300	33	1,055	45	7.3
Pregnant																			
14–18 yr	135	50	530	66	12	1.2	1.2	14	1.6	520	2.2	785	160	23	335	40	1,055	49	10.5
Lactating																			
14–18 yr	160	60	885	96	16	1.2	1.3	13	1.7	450	2.4	985	209	7	300	35	1,055	59	10.9

NOTE: This table presents Estimated Average Requirements (EARs), which serve two purposes: they are used to assess the adequacy of population intakes and as the basis for calculation of the Recommended Dietary Allowances for individuals for those nutrients. EARs have not been established for vitamin D, vitamin K, pantothenic acid, biotin, choline, calcium, chromium, fluoride, manganese, or other nutrients not yet evaluated by the DRI process. CHO = carbohydrates; g/day = grams per day; mg/day = milligrams per day; μg/d = micrograms per day.

[a]As retinol activity equivalents (RAEs). 1 RAE = 1 μg retinol, 12 μg β-carotene, 24 μg α-carotene, or 24 μg β-cryptoxanthin. The RAE for dietary provitamin A carotenoids is two-fold greater than retinol equivalents (RE), whereas the RAE for preformed vitamin A is the same as RE.

[b]As α-tocopherol. α-Tocopherol includes *RRR*-α-tocopherol, the only form of α-tocopherol that occurs naturally in foods, and the *2R*-stereoisomeric forms of α-tocopherol (*RRR*-, *RSR*-, *RRS*-, and *RSS*-α-tocopherol) that occur in fortified foods and supplements. It does not include the *2S*-stereoisomeric forms of α-tocopherol (*SRR*-, *SSR*-, *SRS*-, and *SSS*-α-tocopherol), also found in fortified foods and supplements.

[c]As niacin equivalents; 1 mg of niacin = 60 mg of tryptophan.

[d]As dietary folate equivalents (DFE); 1 DFE = 1 μg food folate = 0.6 μg of folic acid from fortified food or as a supplement consumed with food = 0.5 μg of a supplement taken on an empty stomach.

SOURCE: IOM, 2006.

TABLE K-2 DRIs: Recommended Dietary Allowances and Adequate Intakes, Vitamins

Life-Stage Group	Vitamin A (μg/d)[a]	Vitamin C (mg/d)	Vitamin D (μg/d)[b,c]	Vitamin E (mg/d)[d]	Vitamin K (μg/d)	Thiamin (mg/d)	Ribo-flavin (mg/d)	Niacin (mg/d)[e]	Vitamin B_6 (mg/d)	Folate (μg/d)[f]	Vitamin B_{12} (μg/d)	Panto-thenic Acid (mg/d)	Biotin (μg/d)	Choline (mg/d)[g]
Children														
4–8 yr	**400**	**25**	5*	**7**	55*	**0.6**	**0.6**	**8**	**0.6**	**200**	**1.2**	3*	12*	250*
Males														
9–13 yr	**600**	**45**	5*	**11**	60*	**0.9**	**0.9**	**12**	**1.0**	**300**	**1.8**	4*	20*	375*
14–18 yr	**900**	**75**	5*	**15**	75*	**1.2**	**1.3**	**16**	**1.3**	**400**	**2.4**	5*	25*	550*
Females														
9–13 yr	**600**	**45**	5*	**11**	60*	**0.9**	**0.9**	**12**	**1.0**	**300**	**1.8**	4*	20*	375*
14–18 yr	**700**	**65**	5*	**15**	75*	**1.0**	**1.0**	**14**	**1.2**	**400**[h]	**2.4**	5*	25*	400*
Pregnant														
14–18 yr	**750**	**80**	5*	**15**	75*	**1.4**	**1.4**	**18**	**1.9**	**600**[i]	**2.6**	6*	30*	450*
Lactating														
14–18 yr	**1,200**	**115**	5*	**19**	75*	**1.4**	**1.6**	**17**	**2.0**	**500**	**2.8**	7*	35*	550*

NOTE: This table presents Recommended Dietary Allowances (RDAs) in boldface type and Adequate Intakes (AIs) in ordinary type followed by an asterisk. RDAs and AIs may both be used as goals for individual intakes. An RDA is set to meet the needs of almost all (97 to 98 percent) individuals in a group. It is calculated from an Estimated Average Requirement (EAR). If sufficient scientific evidence is not available to establish an EAR and, thus, to calculate an RDA, an AI is usually developed. For healthy breast-fed infants, the AI is the mean intake. The AI for other life-stage and gender groups is believed to cover the needs of all individuals in the group, but a lack of data or uncertainty in the data prevent the percentage of individuals covered by this intake from being able to be specified with confidence. mg/day = milligrams per day; μg/d = micrograms per day.

[a]As retinol activity equivalents (RAEs). 1 RAE = 1 μg retinol, 12 μg β-carotene, 24 μg α-carotene, or 24 μg β-cryptoxanthin. The RAE for dietary provitamin A carotenoids is twofold greater than the retinol equivalents (RE), whereas the RAE for preformed vitamin A is the same as the RE.

[b]As cholecalciferol. 1 μg cholecalciferol = 40 international units of vitamin D.

[c]In the absence of adequate exposure to sunlight.

[d]As α-tocopherol. α-Tocopherol includes *RRR*-α-tocopherol, the only form of α-tocopherol that occurs naturally in foods, and the *2R*-stereoisomeric forms of α-tocopherol (*RRR*-, *RSR*-, *RRS*-, and *RSS*-α-tocopherol) that occur in fortified foods and supplements. It does not include the *2S*-stereoisomeric forms of α-tocopherol (*SRR*-, *SSR*-, *SRS*-, and *SSS*-α-tocopherol), also found in fortified foods and supplements.

[e]As niacin equivalents (NE); 1 mg of niacin = 60 mg of tryptophan; for ages 0–6 months = preformed niacin (not NE) is counted.

[f]As dietary folate equivalents (DFE); 1 DFE = 1 μg food folate = 0.6 μg of folic acid from fortified food or as a supplement consumed with food = 0.5 μg of a supplement taken on an empty stomach.

[g]Although AIs have been set for choline, there are few data to assess whether a dietary supply of choline is needed at all stages of the life cycle, and it may be that the choline requirement can be met by endogenous synthesis at some of these stages.

[h]In view of evidence linking folate intake with neural tube defects in the fetus, it is recommended that all women capable of becoming pregnant consume 400 micrograms from supplements or fortified foods, in addition to the intake of food folate from a varied diet.

[i]It is assumed that women will continue consuming 400 micrograms from supplements or fortified food until their pregnancy is confirmed and they enter prenatal care, which ordinarily occurs after the end of the periconceptional period—the critical time for the formation of the neural tube.

SOURCE: IOM, 2006.

TABLE K-3 DRIs: Recommended Dietary Allowances and Adequate Intakes, Elements

Life-Stage Group	Calcium (mg/d)	Chromium (µg/d)	Copper (µg/d)	Fluoride (mg/d)	Iodine (µg/d)	Iron (mg/d)	Magnesium (mg/d)	Manganese (mg/d)	Molybdenum (µg/d)	Phosphorus (mg/d)	Selenium (µg/d)	Zinc (mg/d)	Potassium (g/d)	Sodium (g/d)	Chloride (g/d)
Children															
4–8 yr	800*	15*	**440**	1*	**90**	**10**	**130**	1.5*	**22**	**500**	**30**	**5**	3.8*	1.2*	1.9*
Males															
9–13 yr	1,300*	25*	**700**	2*	**120**	**8**	**240**	1.9*	**34**	**1,250**	**40**	**8**	4.5*	1.5*	2.3*
14–18 yr	1,300*	35*	**890**	3*	**150**	**11**	**410**	2.2*	**43**	**1,250**	**55**	**11**	4.7*	1.5*	2.3*
Females															
9–13 yr	1,300*	21*	**700**	2*	**120**	**8**	**240**	1.6*	**34**	**1,250**	**40**	**8**	4.5*	1.5*	2.3*
14–18 yr	1,300*	24*	**890**	3*	**150**	**15**	**360**	1.6*	**43**	**1,250**	**55**	**9**	4.7*	1.5*	2.3*
Pregnant															
14–18 yr	1,300*	29*	**1,000**	3*	**220**	**27**	**400**	2.0*	**50**	**1,250**	**60**	**12**	4.7*	1.5*	2.3*
Lactating															
14–18 yr	1,300*	44*	**1,300**	3*	**290**	**10**	**360**	2.6*	**50**	**1,250**	**70**	**13**	5.1*	1.5*	2.3*

NOTE: This table presents Recommended Dietary Allowances (RDAs) in boldface type and Adequate Intakes (AIs) in ordinary type followed by an asterisk. RDAs and AIs may both be used as goals for individual intakes. An RDA is set to meet the needs of almost all (97 to 98 percent) individuals in a group. It is calculated from an Estimated Average Requirement (EAR). If sufficient scientific evidence is not available to establish an EAR and, thus, to calculate an RDA, an AI is usually developed. For healthy breast-fed infants, the AI is the mean intake. The AI for other life stage and gender groups is believed to cover the needs of all individuals in the group, but a lack of data or uncertainty in the data prevent the percentage of individuals covered by this intake from being able to be specified with confidence. g/d = grams per day; mg/day = milligrams per day; µg/d = micrograms per day.
SOURCE: IOM, 2006.

TABLE K-4 DRIs: Tolerable Upper Intake Levels, Vitamins

Life-Stage Group	Vitamin A (μg/d)[a]	Vitamin C (mg/d)	Vitamin D (μg/d)	Vitamin E (mg/d)[b,c]	Vitamin K (μg/d)	Thiamin (mg/d)	Riboflavin (mg/d)	Niacin (mg/d)[c]	Vitamin B_6 (mg/d)	Folate (μg/d)[c]	Vitamin B_{12} (μg/d)	Pantothenic Acid (mg/d)	Biotin (μg/d)	Choline (mg/d)	Carotenoids[d]
Children															
4–8 yr	900	650	50	300	ND	ND	ND	15	40	400	ND	ND	ND	1.0	ND
Males															
9–13 yr	1,700	1,200	50	600	ND	ND	ND	20	60	600	ND	ND	ND	2.0	ND
14–18 yr	2,800	1,800	50	800	ND	ND	ND	30	80	800	ND	ND	ND	3.0	ND
Females															
9–13 yr	1,700	1,200	50	600	ND	ND	ND	20	60	600	ND	ND	ND	2.0	ND
14–18 yr	2,800	1,800	50	800	ND	ND	ND	30	80	800	ND	ND	ND	3.0	ND
Pregnant															
14–18 yr	2,800	1,800	50	800	ND	ND	ND	30	80	800	ND	ND	ND	3.0	ND
Lactating															
14–18 yr	2,800	1,800	50	800	ND	ND	ND	30	80	800	ND	ND	ND	3.0	ND

NOTE: A Tolerable Upper Intake Level (UL) is the highest level of daily nutrient intake that is likely to pose no risk of adverse health effects to almost all individuals in the general population. Unless otherwise specified, the UL represents total intake from food, water, and supplements. Because of a lack of suitable data, ULs could not be established for vitamin K, thiamin, riboflavin, vitamin B_{12}, pantothenic acid, biotin, and carotenoids. In the absence of a UL, extra caution may be warranted in consuming levels above the recommended intakes. Members of the general population should be advised not to routinely consume amounts in excess of the UL. The UL is not meant to apply to individuals who are treated with the nutrient under medical supervision or to individuals with predisposing conditions that modify their sensitivity to the nutrient. mg/day = milligrams per day; ND = not determinable because of a lack of data on adverse effects in this age group and concern over the lack of an ability to handle excess amounts. The source of the intake should be from food only to prevent high levels of intake; μg/d = micrograms per day.

[a]As preformed vitamin A only.

[b]As α-tocopherol; applies to any form of supplemental α-tocopherol.

[c]The ULs for vitamin E, niacin, and folate apply to synthetic forms obtained from supplements, fortified foods, or a combination of the two.

[d]β-Carotene supplements are advised only to serve as a provitamin A source for individuals at risk of vitamin A deficiency.

SOURCE: IOM, 2006.

TABLE K-5 DRIs: Tolerable Upper Intake Levels, Elements

Life Stage Group	Calcium (g/d)	Chromium	Copper (μg/d)	Fluoride (mg/d)	Iodine (μg/d)	Iron (mg/d)	Magnesium (mg/d)[a]	Manganese (mg/d)	Molybdenum (μg/d)	Phosphorus (g/d)	Potassium	Selenium (μg/d)	Zinc (mg/d)	Sodium (g/d)	Chloride (g/d)
Children															
4–8 yr	2.5	ND	3,000	2.2	300	40	110	3.0	600	3.0	ND	150	12	1.9	2.9
Males															
9–13 yr	2.5	ND	5,000	10	600	40	350	6.0	1,100	4.0	ND	280	23	2.2	3.4
14–18 yr	2.5	ND	8,000	10	900	45	350	9.0	1,700	4.0	ND	400	34	2.3	3.6
Females															
9–13 yr	2.5	ND	5,000	10	600	40	350	6.0	1,100	4.0	ND	280	23	2.2	3.4
14–18 yr	2.5	ND	8,000	10	900	45	350	9.0	1,700	4.0	ND	400	34	2.3	3.6
Pregnant															
14–18 yr	2.5	ND	8,000	10	900	45	350	9.0	1,700	3.5	ND	400	34	2.3	3.6
Lactating															
14–18 yr	2.5	ND	8,000	10	900	45	350	9.0	1,700	4.0	ND	400	34	2.3	3.6

NOTE: A Tolerable Upper Intake Level (UL) is the highest level of daily nutrient intake that is likely to pose no risk of adverse health effects to almost all individuals in the general population. Unless otherwise specified, the UL represents total intake from food, water, and supplements. Because of a lack of suitable data, In the absence of a UL, extra caution may be warranted in consuming levels above the recommended intakes. Members of the general population should be advised not to routinely consume amounts in excess of the UL. The UL is not meant to apply to individuals who are treated with the nutrient under medical supervision or to individuals with predisposing conditions that modify their sensitivity to the nutrient. mg/day = milligrams per day; ND = not determinable because of a lack of data on adverse effects in this age group and concern over the lack of an ability to handle excess amounts. The source of the intake should be from food only to prevent high levels of intake; μg/d = micrograms per day.

[a]The ULs for magnesium represent intake from a pharmacological agent only and do not include intake from food and water.

SOURCE: IOM, 2006.

TABLE K-6 DRIs: Recommended Dietary Allowances and Adequate Intakes, Total Water and Macronutrient

Life-Stage Group	Total Water[a] (L/d)	Carbo-Hydrate (g/d)	Total Fiber (g/d)	Fat (g/d)	Linoleic Acid (g/d)	α-Linoleic Acid (g/d)	Protein[b] (g/d)
Children							
4–8 yr	1.7*	**130**	25*	ND	7*	0.9*	**19**
Males							
9–13 yr	2.4*	**130**	31*	ND	12*	1.2*	**34**
14–18 yr	3.3*	**130**	38*	ND	16*	1.6*	**52**
Females							
9–13 yr	2.1*	**130**	26*	ND	10*	1.0*	**34**
14–18 yr	2.3*	**130**	26*	ND	11*	1.1*	**46**
Pregnant							
14–18 yr	3.0*	**175**	28*	ND	13*	1.4*	**71**
Lactating							
14–18 yr	3.8*	**210**	29*	ND	13*	1.3*	**71**

NOTE: This table presents Recommended Dietary Allowances (RDAs) in boldface type and Adequate Intakes (AIs) in ordinary type followed by an asterisk. RDAs and AIs may both be used as goals for individual intakes. An RDA is set to meet the needs of almost all (97 to 98 percent) individuals in a group. It is calculated from an Estimated Average Requirement (EAR). If sufficient scientific evidence is not available to establish an EAR and, thus, to calculate an RDA, an AI is usually developed. For healthy breast-fed infants, the AI is the mean intake. The AI for other life-stage and gender groups is believed to cover the needs of all individuals in the group, but a lack of data or uncertainty in the data prevent the percentage of individuals covered by this intake from being able to be specified with confidence. g/d = grams per day; L/d = liters per day; ND = not determined.

[a]Total water includes all water contained in food, beverages, and drinking water.

[b]On the basis of the number of grams protein per kilograms of body weight for the reference body weight, for example, for adults 0.8 grams per kilogram of body weight for the reference body weight.

SOURCE: IOM, 2006.

TABLE K-7 Acceptable Macronutrient Distribution Ranges

Macronutrient	Range (percent of energy) for the Following Age Groups[a]: 1–3 yr	4–18 yr
Fat		
n-6 Polyunsaturated fatty acids[b] (linoleic acid)	30–40	25–35
n-3 Polyunsaturated fatty acids[b] (α-linolenic acid)	0.6–1.2	0.6–1.2
Carbohydrate	45–65	45–65
Protein	5–20	10–30

[a]The Acceptable Macronutrient Distribution Range is the percentage of energy intake that is associated with a reduced risk of chronic disease yet that provides adequate amounts of essential nutrients.

[b]Approximately 10 percent of the total can come from longer-chain *n*-3 or *n*-6 fatty acids.

SOURCE: IOM, 2006.

TABLE K-8 Additional Macronutrient Recommendations

Macronutrient	Recommended Intake
Dietary cholesterol	As low as possible while consuming a nutritionally adequate diet
Trans fatty acids	As low as possible while consuming a nutritionally adequate diet
Saturated fatty acids	As low as possible while consuming a nutritionally adequate diet
Added sugars	Limit to a maximum intake of no more than 25% of total energy[a]

[a]Not a recommended intake. A daily intake of added sugars that individuals should aim for to achieve a healthful diet was not set.
SOURCE: IOM, 2006.

TABLE K-9 Estimated Energy Requirements

Group	Equation Used to Estimate Energy Requirement
Males	
3–8 yr	EER = 88.5 – (61.9 × age [yr]) + PA × [(26.7 × weight [kg]) + (903 × height [m])] + 20
9–18 yr	EER = 88.5 – (61.9 × age [yr]) + PA ×[(26.7 × weight [kg]) +(903 × height [m])] + 25
Females	
3–8 yr	EER = 135.3 – (30.8 × age [yr]) + PA × [(10.0 × weight [kg]) + (934 × height [m])] + 20
9–18 yr	EER = 135.3 – (30.8 × age [yr]) + PA × [(10.0 × weight [kg]) + (934 × height [m])] + 25

NOTE: Estimated energy requirement (calories per day) = total energy expenditure + energy deposition; kg = kilograms; m = meters; PA = physical activity coefficient (see Table J-10). These equations provide an estimate of energy requirement. Relative body weight (i.e., loss, stable, gain) is the preferred indicator of energy adequacy.
SOURCE: IOM, 2006.

TABLE K-10 Physical Activity Coefficients for Use in Estimated Energy Requirement Equations

	Physical Activity Coefficients for the Following Levels of Activity:			
	Sedentary (PAL 1.0–1.39)	Low Active (PAL 1.4–1.59)	Active (PAL 1.6–1.89)	Very Active (PAL 1.9–2.5)
Group	Typical daily living activities (e.g., household tasks, walking to the bus)	Typical daily living activities plus 30–60 minutes of daily moderate activity (e.g., walking at 5–7 km/h)	Typical daily living activities plus at least 60 minutes of daily moderate activity	Typical daily living activities plus at least 60 minutes of daily moderate activity plus an additional 60 minutes of vigorous activity or 120 minutes of moderate activity
Males, 3–18 yr	1.00	1.13	1.26	1.42
Females, 3–18 yr	1.00	1.16	1.31	1.56

NOTE: PAL = physical activity level.
SOURCE: IOM, 2006.

Appendix L

MyPyramid Food Intake Pattern Compared with Meal Requirements for the NSLP

This appendix presents a table comparing the amounts of food specified by the MyPyramid food intake pattern with the current school meal requirements for a school lunch. The committee divided the total daily MyPyramid amounts for selected calorie levels by 3 since, by law, school lunch must provide one-third of a day's intake of calories and nutrients.

TABLE L-1 Lunch Pattern Based on 2,400-Calorie MyPyramid Food Intake Pattern Compared with Meal Requirements for the National School Lunch Program

		NSLP Traditional Food-Based Menu Plan		NSLP Enhanced Food-Based Menu Plan	
MyPyramid Food Group	MyPyramid Pattern Divided by 3[a]	Minimum Requirement	Minimum Requirement as a % of One-Third of the MyPyramid Pattern	Minimum Requirement	Minimum Requirement as a % of One-Third of the MyPyramid Pattern
Total fruit (c/meal)	⅔ c	N/S	NA	N/S	NA
Total veg (c/meal)	1 c	N/S	NA	N/S	NA
Total fruit/veg (c/meal)	1 ⅔ c	¾ c	45%	1 c	60%
Dark green veg (c/wk)	1 c	N/S	NA	N/S	NA
Orange veg (c/wk)	⅔c	N/S	NA	N/S	NA
Legumes (c/wk)	1 c	N/S	NA	N/S	NA
Starchy veg (c/wk)	2 c	N/S	NA	N/S	NA
Other veg (c/wk)	2 ⅓ c	N/S	NA	N/S	NA
Total grain (oz eq/meal)	2 ⅔ c	1.6	60%	3	112%
Whole grains (oz eq/meal)	1.3 oz	N/S	NA	N/S	NA
Total milk group (c/meal)	1 c	1 c	100%	1 c	100%
Total meat and bean (oz eq/meal)	2.17 oz	3 oz	138%	2 oz	92%
Oils (tsp/meal)	2 ⅓ tsp	N/S	NA	N/S	NA
Discretionary calorie[b] allowance (calories/meal)	121 calories	N/S	NA	N/S	NA

NOTE: c = c; eq = equivalent; NA = not applicable; N/S = not specified; NSLP = National School Lunch Program; oz = ounce; tsp = teaspoon; veg = vegetable.

[a]Daily recommendations have been divided by 3 for comparison of the values with the current NSLP guidelines for a school lunch (which should provide one-third of a day's intake of calories and nutrients).

[b]Discretionary calories are the calories remaining after the consumption of the calories needed to meet recommended nutrient intakes. These can be used to select foods with higher fat or sugar contents.

SOURCE: Derived from USDA, 2000b, 2005.

Appendix M

Estimation of Cost of Food for One Week's Menu: Example for Elementary School Level

Table M-1 lists an example of lunch menus for a 5-day week for an elementary school selected from the most commonly used school menus reported in the third School Nutrition and Dietary Assessment study (and compiled by Abt Associates for the committee's use). These menus were used to determine the base food costs of a meal.

TABLE M-1 Example Estimation of Cost of Food for Menus for 5 Days at the Elementary School Level

Day of Week and Food Component	Food	Portion Size (grams)	Number of Reimbursable Servings	Food Cost ($) per Pound in 1996–1997*	Food Cost ($) per Serving in 1996–1997*
Monday (245 reimbursable meals served)					
Milk	Milk, cow's, fluid, 1% fat	244.0	55	0.29	0.156
Milk	Milk, cow's, fluid, skim or nonfat	245.0	13	0.29	0.157
Milk	Milk, chocolate, low-fat milk based	249.6	177	0.30	0.165
Fruit/vegetable	Applesauce, stewed apples, with sugar	95.6	82	0.38	0.080
Fruit/vegetable	Peach, cooked or canned, in light or medium syrup	94.1	21	0.59	0.122
Fruit/vegetable	Orange juice, canned/bottled/carton, unsweetened	249.0	95	0.44	0.242
Fruit/vegetable	Hash brown patties (school service)	54.0	245	0.43	0.051
Combination entrée	Burrito with beans and cheese (school service)	150.3	63	1.13	0.374
Meat/meat alternate	Pork sausage, fresh, bulk, patty or link, cooked	56.0	182	1.72	0.212
Bread/grain	French toast sticks (school service)	113.4	146	1.30	0.325
Other	Cheese, mozzarella, part skim (including low fat)	28.4	150	1.90	0.119
Condiments	Tomato catsup	30.0	233	0.71	0.047
Toppings or spreads	Pancake syrup, nfs	59.1	143	0.49	0.064
Average cost of meal served					**0.947**
Tuesday (244 reimbursable meals served)					
Milk	Milk, cow's, fluid, 1% fat	244.0	44	0.29	0.156
Milk	Milk, cow's, fluid, skim or nonfat	245.0	14	0.29	0.157
Milk	Milk, chocolate, low-fat milk based	249.6	185	0.30	0.165
Fruit/vegetable	Applesauce, stewed apples, with sugar	95.6	57	0.38	0.080
Fruit/vegetable	Pear, cooked or canned, in light syrup	93.4	81	0.64	0.132
Fruit/vegetable	Celery, raw (include celery, nfs)	24.8	106	0.40	0.022
Fruit/vegetable	Carrots, raw	24.4	106	1.06	0.057

TABLE M-1 Example Estimation of Cost of Food for Menus for 5 Days at the Elementary School Level

Day of Week and Food Component	Food	Portion Size (grams)	Number of Reimbursable Servings	Food Cost ($) per Pound in 1996–1997*	Food Cost ($) per Serving in 1996–1997*
Combination entrée	Frankfurter or hot dog, plain, on bun	85.0	113	1.19	0.223
Combination entrée	Spaghetti with tomato sauce and meatballs	271.1	78	1.22	0.729
Condiments	Creamy dressing, with sour cream/buttermilk and oil	22.0	106	0.55	0.027
Condiments	Tomato catsup	60.0	96	0.71	0.094
Average cost of meal served					**0.644**
Wednesday (247 reimbursable meals served)					
Milk	Milk, cow's, fluid, 1% fat	244.0	9	0.29	0.156
Milk	Milk, cow's, fluid, skim or nonfat	245.0	13	0.29	0.157
Milk	Milk, chocolate, low-fat milk based	249.6	206	0.30	0.165
Fruit/vegetable	Banana, raw	56.3	144	0.38	0.047
Fruit/vegetable	Raisins (include cinnamon-coated raisins)	24.1	52	1.69	0.090
Fruit/vegetable	Corn, yellow, cooked, from canned, fat added	63.4	167	0.39	0.054
Combination entrée	Pizza sticks or dippers (school service)	109.4	130	1.53	0.369
Combination entrée	Pizza with sausage, thin crust	134.7	103	1.21	0.359
Condiments	Tomato sauce	91.9	142	0.32	0.065
Average cost of meal served					**0.616**
Thursday (246 reimbursable meals served)					
Milk	Milk, cow's, fluid, 1% fat	244.0	45	0.29	0.156
Milk	Milk, cow's, fluid, skim or nonfat	245.0	18	0.29	0.157
Milk	Milk, chocolate, low-fat milk based	249.6	183	0.30	0.165
Fruit/vegetable	Banana, raw	56.3	23	0.38	0.047

TABLE M-1 Example Estimation of Cost of Food for Menus for 5 Days at the Elementary School Level

Day of Week and Food Component	Food	Portion Size (grams)	Number of Reimbursable Servings	Food Cost ($) per Pound in 1996–1997*	Food Cost ($) per Serving in 1996–1997*
Fruit/vegetable	Peach, cooked or canned, in light or medium syrup	94.1	69	0.59	0.122
Fruit/vegetable	White potato, complete dry mix, mashed, made with water	113.5	228	0.89	0.223
Meat/meat alternate	Turkey, light and dark meat, roasted, ns as to skin	67.5	146	1.15	0.171
Meat/meat alternate	Breaded beef patty (school service)	113.4	66	1.42	0.355
Bread/grain	Roll, wheat or cracked wheat	56.7	206	1.01	0.126
Dessert	Fruit juice bar, frozen, flavor other than orange	67.1	238	0.86	0.127
Condiments	Tomato catsup	30.0	32	0.71	0.047
Toppings or spreads	Gravy, poultry	29.8	228	1.97	0.129
Average cost of meal served					**0.959**
Friday (235 reimbursable meals served)					
Milk	Milk, cow's, fluid, 1% fat	244.0	47	0.29	0.156
Milk	Milk, cow's, fluid, skim or nonfat	245.0	13	0.29	0.157
Milk	Milk, chocolate, low-fat-milk based	249.6	176	0.30	0.165
Fruit/vegetable	Peach, cooked or canned, in light or medium syrup	94.1	21	0.59	0.122
Fruit/vegetable	Pineapple, cooked or canned, juice pack	93.4	92	0.58	0.119
Fruit/vegetable	Tater tots (school service)	64.0	178	0.43	0.061
Combination entrée	Pizza, cheese, thin crust (school service)	134.7	162	1.21	0.359
Combination entrée	Beef barbecue sandwich or sloppy joe, on bun with beef crumble	156.7	65	3.52	1.216
Bread/grain	Bread, sweet potato with vegetable oil, nfs (include oil, nfs)	28.4	167	0.84	0.053
Condiments	Tomato catsup	30.0	192	0.71	0.047
Average cost of meal served					**0.927**

TABLE M-1 Example Estimation of Cost of Food for Menus for 5 Days at the Elementary School Level

Day of Week and Food Component	Food	Portion Size (grams)	Number of Reimbursable Servings	Food Cost ($) per Pound in 1996–1997*	Food Cost ($) per Serving in 1996–1997*
Weekly means (1996–1997 dollars)	Unweighted				
	Weighted				**0.818**
	July 1996 adjusted to 2006 (July) by CPI (FAFH)**				**1.069**
	July 1996 adjusted to 2008 (July) by CPI (FAFH)**				**1.158**

NOTE: CPI = Consumer Price Index; FAFH = food away from home.
SOURCES: * = USDA, 1998b; ** = U.S. Bureau of Labor Statistics, 2008.